Yoga for Teens

Shawna Schenk

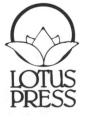

LOTUS
PRESS
PO Box 325
Twin Lakes, WI

HEALTHY LIVING/YOGA/INSPIRATIONAL/TEENAGERS

Photo credit: Mandy Downs

Models: Mia Uranga, Joyce Varias, Jaden Uranga

Printed in the United States of America

Disclaimer: This book, in no way, claims to force any activities on any individual or claim to cure any mental or physical issue. This book is merely inspiration and the activities and advice is given is to be taken by the reader's own choice.

ISBN: 978-0-9406-7634-3

Library of Congress Number: 2015959723

Published by:

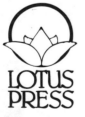

LOTUS
PRESS

Lotus Press
P.O. Box 325
Twin Lakes, WI 53181 USA
800-824-6396 (toll free order phone)
262-889-8561 (office phone)
262-889-2461 (office fax)
www.LotusPress.com (website)
lotuspress@lotuspress.com (email)
Printed In USA

dedicated to...

you, the reader

(because more mentally and physically healthy teens makes for the likelihood of more mentally and physically healthy adults which makes for the likelihood of a more mentally and physically healthy future)

Table of Contents

Preface

Teens and Depression

Yoga teaches you to be honest with yourself: your feelings, your surroundings, your beliefs, your thoughts, and your life. Then, it uses this honesty to help make this world a more honest place. For this reason, this book holds pure and raw honesty from cover to cover.

As a teen, people weren't always honest with me. They either thought I was "too young" to understand the truth, or they were trying to "protect" me. All this did was frustrate me, and falsely prepared me for the "real world." This turned me into a scared young adult who learned a lot about life the hard way. Because of this, I and this book will never do that to you.

This book explains what yoga is and how teens can use yoga to help make their life more peaceful and happy. Maybe you heard of yoga before or you've done it before. This book will show you that yoga is not simply stretch pants and stretching. It is a way to get to know yourself, and then become the best version of yourself, honestly.

The teenage years of life are so amazing, but they are also hard. There are pressures, expectations, and false definitions that hold teens back from being who they truly are. Teens experience lots of growing pains. I know, as a teenager, you are in this phase of life where you are ready to be free, but you still have lots of rules to follow.

I am not a teenager now, but I was one. I didn't learn yoga until I was about 26 years old, and when I learned it, it changed my life for the better. Everyone should have the opportunity to live a better life, so this is part of the reason why I wrote this book for teens on yoga.

I am an adult, and I am a yoga teacher in California. I teach yoga to all types of people. I've literally taught yoga to people from all over the world (from New Jersey to Germany to Jamaica to other countries you only hear about in your history classes). I've taught yoga to happy people and sad people, people who are sick and people who are healthy. I've taught yoga to children as small as two and adults as old as 93. I've taught yoga to people who couldn't understand me (they spoke another language), and I've taught yoga to people who couldn't get out of a chair. Sometimes I even try to teach my dogs yoga. They actually do have a pretty impressive Downward Facing Dog!

I also teach people to be yoga teachers. I teach adults how to teach yoga, and I teach teenagers how to teach yoga to other teens and young kids. I know the majority of your life centers around learning and school, and you have some teachers you don't like, but all teachers are important, and learning never ends. In fact, learning is what keeps this world alive. I am a teacher and student for life.

I went to college and have a bunch of degrees including a Master's degree in Writing, and undergraduate degrees in Early Childhood Education and Sociology. These fancy degrees also helped me understand teens, teaching, and the world.

From this knowledge and experience, I've learned a lot. So here's the honest truth: **All people have problems. Life is about dealing with problems. Teenagers and tweens will have problems, but these problems become magnified because teens are still learning the correct way to deal with their emotions. This is a hard thing to learn and takes time. When emotions are not properly handled, they escalate quickly and can turn into big problems like depression.**

For years, adults believed kids couldn't get depressed! I think this is unbelievable as anyone with a brain can get depressed. Findings are now showing that adults are realizing that it's a real problem. Eleven percent of teens will have a depressive disorder by the age of 18 (NIMH, 2015). I'm not talking about being really sad. I'm talking can't-get-out-of-bed-want-think-about-killing-your-self-depressed. In my opinion, that number is way too high, and there is a reason for it.

One hundred percent of teens do feel sad, angry, mad - all sorts of negative emotions. Not knowing how to cope with them definitely helps lead to consistent depression.

This is not fully your fault. Adults have no problem teaching Math and Science, and although this is changing, many adults and school systems don't teach students all the ways to handle their emotions!

Emotions are new to growing children and teens. Just as you are taught Math, you need to be taught how to deal with feelings. In my opinion, a person who gets an A+ on handling emotions is far more successful in life than a person who get straight A's in Math, Science, History, and English. I got A's and B's in high school, but if here was a subject on coping with my emotions, I'd totally get a D.

Emotions improperly handled can lead to a lot of things like drug use, alcohol use, and the abuse of the respect of sex and your physical body. As a teen, I did these things, too because I didn't know how to handle my negative emotions and the peer pressures around me., Unfortunately, all this did was make me an anxious adult who dealt with panic and worry every day for a long time.

Although I am not a teen, I know this stuff still exists, and is actually arguably worse than it was when I was in high school.

- By the age of 18, 70 percent of teens have had at least one drink of alcohol (TooSmartToStart.org, 2015).

- More than 60 percent of teens admitted that drugs were used, kept, and sold at their schools (DoSomething.org, 2015).

- By the 8th grade, 28 percent of adolescents have consumed alcohol, 15 percent have smoked cigarettes, and 16.5 percent have used marijuana (DoSomething.org, 2015).

- Seventy-one percent of 19 year olds have had sex. (Guttmatcher.org. 2015)

I know I did these things as a teen, too because I didn't know otherwise. These things were "fun" and everyone was doing them.

As an adult, looking back, I realize these dangerous activities are more than that. They provide a mask: a way to not have to deal with growing up or any negative emotions that teens feel.

Lots of teens drink alcohol, have sex before they are ready, and do drugs to deal with depression. The important thing here to remember is that, ironically, these outlets don't deal with these emotions, but instead make them worse. Pushing away or masking feelings is not a game. Depression is not a joke. It can lead to death. (NAMI.org, 2015)

- The third leading cause of death of teens aged 12-18 is suicide.

- Eighteen million teens have thought of killing themselves.

- Every day 5,400 teens attempt suicide.

I'm going to stop throwing numbers at you. I know you know I know this stuff is going on. I also know it is probably your first instinct to lie about it or hide it from adults. But as adults, we've been there, so we know what is going on.

Plus, the statistics show it. This stuff is real, this stuff is going on, and most likely you have experienced on or more of these things, or you've been surrounded by it.

Awareness is key: from this awareness change can happen. As an adult, I learned that yoga taught me how to change, and how to deal with my emotions properly and live peacefully. I changed so much that I changed my career and made it my job to help others.

Teenagers have a lot of love, understanding, and knowledge. Ninety-six and one-half percent of teenagers have performed random acts of kindness to strangers (Stageoflife.org, 2015).

This proves that more than all the bad stuff, teens are and do good stuff! You guys are amazing. I can't even tell you how many adults would never perform a random act of kindness. I believe this is because they are so overburdened by negative emotions they have never properly dealt with over the years and years of their life.

Yoga may be a way to help you help others. Because I am yoga a teacher, I know a lot about yoga, and I am going to explain a lot of this knowledge to you in this book. Also, because I used to be a teenager I've experienced a lot of things that you have.

I know what it's like to feel ugly, to have a crush on someone who doesn't even know you exist, and to be obsessed with being in love. I know what it's like to want to get kissed so badly. I know what it's like to be curious and super confused with sex and being naked. I lost my virginity when I was 17, and it was nothing like the movies. It was a pretty weird experience, and I wish I would have waited.

I know what it is like to want to be free. I know what is like to feel like I know everything and no one can teach me anything; to "hate" my parents and teachers, to get grounded over something I think is "stupid." I know what it's like to be a brat, to have my first heartbreak, to get in trouble in school for saying a bad word or writing notes to my friends instead of taking notes in Spanish (which would really help me now as an adult when I go down to Mexico!).

I remember how awesome it was to learn to drive! I remember how excited I was to hang out with my first boyfriend. I remember how I thought my life was over when he dumped me.

I also know what it's like to want to be accepted. I remember the cliques in school. I remember not joining the band because it was for "dorks" (but deep down I really wished I knew how to play an instrument). I had my first taste of alcohol when I was teen. I pretended to like it to fit in, but it was disgusting and actually hurt my throat.

I remember wanting to spend all of my money on the coolest clothes, and getting ready for school was one of the most important things. I remember "hating" other girls and boys. I remember wanting to be other girls.

I **remember stress**: it was so important to be "good" in school and "good" in sports and join lots of clubs. I remember feeling tired and overworked, but doing it because I thought I had to. I know how much pressure there is to get good grades, study really hard for tests, take boring, long SAT classes, and try to figure out what I wanted to be when I grew up. I also know what it's like to be so confused and pressured when it came to figuring out what college I wanted to go to.

There are a lot of things, though, that you are experiencing today that I never did. In fact, cell phones just started to get popular when I was 17, and the internet was brand new at this time too (you're totally thinking I'm ancient. Don't worry, I will reveal my age later on in this book). I know what it's like to be a teen, but I don't know what it is like to be you, or to be a teen living in today's world.

Honestly, yoga has taught me that all people are the same, no matter what age they are. Everyone wants the same thing: love and peace, and most of us have no clue how to get it, so our life is blurred up with anger, depression, and fear.

Because I will always be honest with you, and I can't pretend to be a teenager like you are, there are also stories and art work from other teenagers in this book. They may be your age (or around your age) and some of them teach or do yoga. They, too, understand you.

On a side note: I want to tell you if you want a story of yours in this book or on my webpage, please email it to me. Your words are important as are your stories! The more teens talking to teens about emotions in a healthy and honest way, the better the world will be, so email a story or art work: info@YogaWithShawna.com

Be sure to get your parent's permission first though (I know, one of the "problems" of being a teen-asking your parents about everything, but trust me, they are smarter than you give them credit for, and they only want what is best for you.) Also, check out www.YogaWithShawna.com for other teen yoga stories and art.

Yoga For Teens

Chapter 1

Yoga for Peace

What is yoga?
Yoga is a practice which helps people gain awareness of their body and mind. It teaches different ways to bring mental and physical health to a person. Its main focus is to make a person's mind and body strong, healthy, and peaceful.

Yoga is over 5,000 years old and was started in India. We know this because of writings that archaeologists have discovered and traditions that Indians have passed down for thousands of years.

Of the many sacred writings, one of the best known texts is called, *The Yoga Sutras*. *The Yoga Sutras* explain what yoga is and how to do it. This text was written in Sanskrit, which is the classical language of India. If you ever took a yoga class and heard a teacher say a funny name, it was most likely a Sanskrit word. Many teachers and texts use some Sanskrit when discussing yoga. This is to honor the past history of yoga.

Yoga is not a religion. Some people confuse yoga with religion because it was started in a religious country. Yoga does not ask you to pray or honor any god or deity (religious figure). All it asks is that you develop a strong relationship with yourself. Sometimes when this happens, you start to develop a spiritual side.

Spirituality is different from religion because, although both center on a belief system, spirituality allows you to define your own belief system. Unlike religion, there is no organization or group telling you what is "right" and what you should believe. Instead, through establishing a relationship with your mind and body, you are able to establish a belief system of your own. This belief system may be the same or different than another person's. It may even bring you to a connection with your soul.

The *Yoga Sutras* were written by Patanjali. Patanjali is not a person. It is a Sanskrit word which can be translated to "wise man" or "important author." Because yoga has been passed down for thousands of years, there is not just one person who "wrote" this text; Patanjali is the name used to represent all of the contributors of this important, yogic book.

"Yoga" is also a Sanskirt word. It means "to unite" or "to join" Based on this translation, the focus of yoga is to unite awareness with yourself. You want to try your best to join your mind, body, and soul with the world around you.

The Yoga Sutras defines yoga in eight different ways. There are eight limbs (or parts) of yoga. Just as a tree has many limbs or branches, one branch is not more important than another. All of the branches on a tree are equally important as they all help the tree stand tall, give shelter and shade to other animals, bring food to humans, bugs, and animals, and bring beauty and inspiration to the world.

The eight limbs of yoga are the same as the branches on a tree. Not one branch of yoga is better or more important than another. All the branches of yoga contribute to the end result of yoga which is peace. We need to practice them all.

The First Limb
The first limb of yoga is called the "Yamas." "Yamas" is a Sanskrit word. The "yamas" are five rules that help you be good to other people and this world.

The first "Yama" is "Ahimsa," which means "kindness." You first practice yoga by being kind to all people, even those people who are not very nice. Yoga believes if you are nice to everyone, you will be less likely to get angry or upset, and this will allow you to be a happier and healthier person.

The second "Yama" is "Satya," which means "truthfulness." Yoga teaches us that it is important to always tell the truth (and do it in a kind way—remember Ahimsa.) By being honest, you are not hiding anything. When you hide something, it can cause you stress which can make you very unhappy.

The third "Yama" is "Asteya," which means "nonstealing." Yoga reminds us to not take anything that is not ours. Imagine if your best friend stole your boyfriend or girlfriend. That wouldn't feel very good. Lots of people steal, but yoga reminds us to "be the change," by not taking anything that doesn't belong to us. This means it doesn't matter if you are stealing a pencil or a bike. Taking from others takes from all the goodness that you have inside of you.

The fourth "Yama" is "Brahmacarya," which teaches the importance of honoring your body. This honor is especially important when talking about sex and kissing and touching other's bodies. Kissing and sex are topics all teens need to talk about. Sex is a big responsibility and, if not done safely, there are a lot of consequences.

Yoga discusses the importance of not using physical touch for anything other than a way to connect with your spiritual self.

Connecting with the spiritual self takes time. First, you must establish a strong physical and emotional relationship; getting to know who you really are. Because this is really confusing, especially as a teenager who doesn't have complete independence, sex is not something teens should be having or doing.

Instead, Brahmacarya teaches teens the importance of getting to know themselves and respecting their mind and body. Your body is a temple: it should be honored and respected. It is not a place to let others in freely. Lots of adults still don't understand this, and it leads them to big trouble.

The fifth "Yama" is "Aparigraha," which means "non-greediness." It is so very important to be a selfless, giving person. Yoga teaches the importance of sharing what you have with others. This means to take only what you need and dedicate time to give to others. When you give to others you set an example for others to be givers too. Money is not as important as being giving and fair to other people. Helping others is what brings peace and harmony in this world.

The Second Limb

The second limb of yoga is called the "Niyamas." The Yamas talk about being a good person to the world, while the Niyamas talk about being a good person to yourself. It is so important to be good to yourself. The Niyamas list five rules for healthy, self-care.

The first "Niyama" is "Sauca," which means "cleanliness." It is important to keep your inner and outer self clean. This means not only washing your body and brushing your teeth every day, but it also means wearing clean clothes and keeping your things nice and tidy.

Aside from keeping the outside of our body and our things clean, it is also very important to keep your inside clean. Yoga teaches this! This means eating healthy foods and doing exercise (like the yoga stretches we will talk about in the third limb!). It is also really important to have clean, happy thoughts so this is why we use yoga to remove stress from our life caused by not-so-happy thoughts.

The second "Niyama" is "Santosa," which is translated to mean "contentment." A big part of taking care of yourself is being content and grateful for your life and in your life. Contentment is different from happiness. Life may not always be sunshine and butterflies. Contentment teaches us to be "ok" even when things don't seem ok.

This is a hard concept to understand, especially if something in your life doesn't seem fair or happy. Yoga is a practice, so practicing contentment takes time. The secret of being content all the time is to be grateful.

Be small and simple with your gratitude. If your parents are making you angry, step back and realize what you do have: parents! In the same way, if someone is picking on you, be grateful for the experience, as you are able to become a stronger, more loving person from it. When a person is content all of the time, they are able to be happier more easily, and happiness links to a healthier body and mind. This is such an important thing to learn to prepare you for adulthood.

The third "Niyama" is "Tapas," which means "self-discipline." Another important part of taking care of yourself is being disciplined in your actions; this means being sure to do what you say you are going to do.

Tapas also relates to laziness. Sure, you could sit and play on Instagram® or SnapChat® for hours, but how is that making your body and mind as healthy as it could be? if say you read an inspirational book outside or did some sort of physical activity instead (and kept on the online surfing to a few minutes)?

The fourth "Niyama" is "Svadhyaya." Svadhyaya encourages a person to study themselves. For example, understanding what stresses you out and what makes you happy. You are your own best friend. You will have boyfriends and girlfriends and lots of friends throughout your life, but no one will love you like you will!

Yoga teaches the importance of getting to know yourself better than you know anything or anyone. From this, you can use your knowledge to help make you a better person every day. If, for example, something stresses you out, remove that from your life and replace it with something or someone who relaxes you. Or if it is something you can't remove (like your Math teacher) then practice contentment and gratitude for the moment! (Math will help you as an adult when you are buying things and saving money!).

The fifth "Niyama" is "Isvara-pranidhana" which talks about surrender. There are many, many things in life you cannot control: like how a person acts towards you or what time you have to be home on the weekends. But Isvara-pranidhana reminds you to take care of yourself by surrendering. Do not worry about things you cannot control: there is purpose behind it and everything will be ok (I promise!).

The Third Limb
The third limb is the "Asanas." Asana is Sanskrit for "postures." This is the part of yoga that is the most popular in the United States. It's the fun stuff you do with your body like Dancer's Pose or Splits or Headstands!

It is important to physically move and stretch your body. The asanas or yoga postures do different jobs that work on making your body stronger and your tension less. They help build the strength of all of your organs, blood, cells, joints, and all of the other parts of your body that you probably learned about in health class! They help detox your body (cleaning it to keep it free from sickness). They work hard to remove any tightness or anything in your body that doesn't feel as good as it should. They also work to make your body always feel good and prevent it from future sickness.

Remember when we talked about the tree and all of its branches being important? It is important to remember this: when you do yoga, it doesn't mean you are doing it just by taking a cool picture of yourself doing a backbend! Instead, this is just one part of yoga.

It's really important that you move your body and make it flexible and physically strong every day (that's why we practice headstands and splits!) but it is also important to be a good person to the world and yourself and the other limbs we haven't talked about yet.

Always remember that yoga is not just done on a mat: it's done all the time because its purpose is to make you feel good all of the time!

The Fourth Limb
The fourth limb is "Pranayama," which means "breathing." I think it's really cool that teens do yoga. As I said before, I didn't start doing yoga until I was about 26, and I felt like I learned a lot of stuff in my life (I had a master's degree in college!) but I never learned how to breathe properly. Yoga teaches the importance of breathing.

The breath is something you do every second of every day—it is your "medicine." It makes your body healthy and your mind calm. Most people don't take long enough breaths though! This means our bodies aren't as strong or calm as they could be.

Yoga teaches us how to breathe strong and how to use this breathing every second by explaining different breathing exercises. Many of these breathing exercises will be discussed in this book!

The next four branches of yoga focus all on meditating!
Meditating is difficult for people of all ages to do, so yoga teaches some tricks to get your mind still and focused. It is sort of easy to keep your mind focused when you are doing something fun like watching a movie or hanging with your friends. But it gets harder when you are reading a book that you're not interested in or just hanging out with yourself thinking about something else in your head that already happened or that might happen one day.

Focus will make you better at school, sports, and even all the boring things you have to do even though you don't want to! Keeping focused will make you smarter and more attentive. You also will make better decisions and be less likely to make a mistake. Meditating will also help you be happier and worry less. We all think a lot. Sometimes we think too much. Meditation helps us slow down all the thoughts in our head so we aren't thinking so much, but living our life instead.

A bunch of meditation exercises will be provided in this book, too focused on these next four limbs.

The Fifth Limb
The fifth limb is "Pratyahara," which is one meditation trick to help you calm your mind. It has to do with controlling your senses. The first thing you want to do to stay focused and present is to remove all of those things that distract you. This means not letting your senses take control of your thoughts! For example, if you are studying for a test in the kitchen, and your mom is cooking dinner, you're going to be distracted by the smell of the food and not want to focus on the studying. To practice this limb, you can physically move, but yoga teaches how to shift your focus so you don't even notice your outside surroundings.

Shifting your focus takes a lot of mind control and maturity, but when you practice Pratyahara you will start to be more focused and less distracted! This is really helpful with people with ADD (like myself).

The Sixth Limb
Sometimes you can't remove yourself from distractions: for example, if the boy or girl you like sits in front of you in your boring History class, or all of your friends are around you in this class and all you want to do is talk to them, it may seem impossible to focus. The sixth limb, "Dharana", helps with this!

"Dharana" means concentration. Just like when you concentrate really hard when you are taking a test, concentration or focus will help you meditate and stay present in your life.

To do it, just try your hardest to focus your attention on what is going on in front of you. Our world is so full of distractions (for example,we are always playing on our phone or using some other electronic device like video games or the computer to distract us from the present moment), this can be hard to do. Don't worry, though: it's a practice, so just keep practicing paying attention to what is happening around you and not distracting yourself with other things.

The Seventh Limb
The seventh limb is "Dhyana," which is translated to "observation and reflection." Understanding what meditation is can be tricky because it is so many things, and it's not very easy. You can meditate by sitting, standing, or even moving. As long as you are able to observe your actions and reflect as you are doing it, you are practicing Dhyana.

If you fall asleep when you are meditating or you start to think about other things rather than observing the present moment, it's ok. Use this knowledge of what happened when you tried to meditate, and learn from it! For example, if you tried to meditate and you keep thinking about which college you will go to, then you know that this is what is on the front of your mind, so you should talk about it with others and come up with a plan to make your thoughts a reality. Ultimately, the goal is to stay awake and not let your mind wander off to other thoughts than what is going on right in the present moment.

The Eighth Limb
The eighth limb is called "Samadhi," and this is the place in your mind where you are completely peaceful. It happens when you are not thinking about anything, you are not distracted with anything, and you are truly able to be in the present moment. When this happens, time flies! You also feel calm and this calmness brings bliss. Bliss is better than being happy: it's the feeling you get that lets you know everything is always going to be ok!

Feeling Samdhai is my favorite part of yoga, but getting there takes the other branches. When I'm good to myself and the world, my mind is not distracted. When my body is physically balanced from stretching and moving through the poses, my mind can actively rest. When I pay attention to my breath, it allows me to stay focused, and from all of this, I am able to feel complete bliss! It is pretty cool. Practicing all of the limbs will help you get there.

The Chakras

Another part of yoga is paying attention to energy.
Energy is everywhere, and it affects our body and mind. You know that feeling you get when you walk into a place that makes you happy? That is energy. Now think about a feeling you get when you walk into a crazy place. That is energy, too. The Chakras help define or classify this feeling of energy. They refer to the seven different areas of the body that are affected by energy. Remember energy can be positive or negative.

Chakra Chart

The Chakras	Cause for Negative Energy
Root Chakra (The Muladhara) This energy center is located from the base of the spine all the way down to your feet. When it is in a positive state, your body feels good in this area, and you are really present, focused, and have a happy and stress-free home, school, family, and friend life. You also don't worry about money or having or getting stuff (anything that costs money)!	• parent's divorce • moving • problems at home • school problems • family problems • friend problems • being materialistic • work problems • being too busy • being bored • daydreaming • acting like a brat • money problems • spending too much time indoors • spending too much time on your phone or social media

The Chakras	Cause for Negative Energy
Sacral Chakra (The Svadhisthana) This chakra is located right below the belly button, and it affects all the organs relating to reproduction (except for in males—that's the root chakra) and keeping your body clean like the liver, kidney, intestines, colon, etc. When this chakra is in a positive state of energy, these organs feel and work good, and you are able to go with the flow, be passionate and create! Because this area is linked to reproductive organs, it relates to sex and relationships too!	• sex pressures • sex confusions • sex problems • not going with the flow • being stuck in situations you don't want to • disliking and not accepting your responsibilities • lack of creativity • writer's block (getting stuck when you have to do something creative) • not being inspired • fear • being anal/type A person (not able to accept changes) • PMS

The Chakras	Cause for Negative Energy
Naval Chakra (The Manipura) This energy center relates to your stomach and spleen which is connected to our ego! Did you ever get that feeling of butterflies in your stomach? That's energy. When we are feeling confident, this energy is working right (you won't get butterflies then)!	• nerves before big events • worries about the future • confidence issues • body image issues • shyness • being a "show off" • starting fights • being violent to yourself or others • anger • defensiveness • frustration • agitation • not believing in yourself • being a troublemaker

The Chakras	Cause for Negative Energy
Heart Chakra (The Anahata) This energy is located in your heart, lungs, your circulation, and your shoulders, arms, hands, and fingers. It is positive when we are loving to ourselves and others. You know why lovers hold hands? It's because their heart chakras are touching!	• break ups • bullying • cliques • jealousy • obsession • being mean • dating problems • secret crushes • cheating • making fun of others

The Chakras	Cause for Negative Energy
Throat Chakra (The Visshuddha) This energy is located at the throat, but also affects all of the senses. When it is positive, you are saying, hearing, feeling, seeing, and being everything that is truly you!	• telling lies • gossiping • talking too much • not saying what you want • shyness • being too quiet • not listening • being a "people pleaser" • not doing what you want to do • not showing your true colors • being too loud • being too opinionated • being a "chameleon"

The Chakras	Cause for Negative Energy
Third Eye (The Anja Chakra) There is a little gland, known as the spiritual gland: the Pineal Gland, located on the brain, straight back from the middle of the eyebrows. This chakra is called the "third eye." This is in a positive place when you can trust everything you feel (but can't prove!). You know that gut feeling you get about things? That's your third eye!	• not trusting yourself • not going with your instinct • not listening to your inner wisdom • being delusional • being gullible **Note**: We have two eyes that look out into the world and a third eye—that looks back at us. This eye shows us all of the things inside of us we need to see. Science has shown that this is connected through the Pineal Gland: this gland gets "frozen" from drinking unfiltered water and eating bad foods, so it works its best in kids and teens who haven't had decades of bad food and water! Science shows it doesn't start to get frozen until around age 11 or so…but it can become "unfrozen" if you eat right, avoid fluoride in your toothpaste, and drink clean water. **Don't worry**: "frozen" just means calcified (glands are made of water) which can't hurt you, but will make you less likely to trust your instincts. Kids and teens are super wise because they have this connection with their third eye. Adults are more skeptical in believing in stuff like this: this is because of calcification! So take care of your third eye by eating and drinking right.

The Chakras	Cause for Negative Energy
Crown Chakra (The Sahasrara) This is the energy located on the top of your head! It is connected to your brain and your thoughts. It is in a positive place when you are a believer! It doesn't matter what you believe in—you can even believe in nothing, you just need to believe. having confusions with faith	• having confusions with faith • believing in what others tell you to believe/not having your own belief system • being overly obsessive with your beliefs • being obsessive with your thoughts • not being focused/ having scattered beliefs • being closed-minded

How do I do yoga?

If you are confused on how to actually do yoga—don't worry. You do yoga by practicing one or all of the eight limbs and Chakras just mentioned. Remember the importance of practice. No one is perfect, so take your time. Maybe one day it's really hard for you to focus and meditate, but the next day it could be super easy.

The limbs teach us that yoga is done everywhere! Some yoga is done on a yoga mat and other yoga is done in your everyday life. You physically do yoga through stretching, meditating, and breathing, and you can also do yoga every second by being kind, honest, fair, respectful, and giving to other people and things, and being clean, disciplined, aware and devoted to yourself.

A person who does yoga is known as a "yogi." Yoga is not a "cool club" that you have to be accepted in to or a sport you need to try out or compete for. Anyone can be a yogi. It does not matter what age you are or where you are from. It does not matter if you are a boy or a girl. Yoga is taught in basically every language in this world. It is universal. This is because yoga teaches us that we are all the same. This means we are all equal, and we all deserve physical and mental peace.

Yogis sometimes make mistakes. This is ok! Yogis are human. True yogis work every day to do the best they can to take care of their body and mind.

This book will teach you yoga by explaining how to do different stretches, meditations, and breathing exercises to help deal with your emotions. Yogis often use props when they do certain poses and exercises so the use of props will be given in this book, too. Props are important because they are helpful objects that support you to get stronger and deeper in the pose. There are a number of props you can use to help you (you may want to go to the store and get them).

Here is a quick reference list:

Blocks: Like large foam or wood bricks, blocks are helpful as they bring the ground closer to you! They can help you reach more forward or stretch straighter, which is so important in getting the maximum benefits in many of the poses.

Straps: As a long and skinny piece of fabric (similar to a belt), straps are helpful as an extension of your arms, so you can reach deeper in backbend or further in a leg stretch.

Bolsters: A bolster is a big, firm pillow. Not only is it super comfortable to lay on (which helps you be more still in poses), it can hold you in different poses to help make the pose more accessible.

Blankets: A blanket can be used in a transitional way (especially when laying on your back and meditating) to keep you warm, but if you roll it up like a burrito, you can use to assist you in backbends. You can also fold it into a little pillow and rest on it. Remember, the aim of yoga is to feel so comfortable you could fall asleep, but you don't because you are conscious and aware.

Many stores sell "special yoga versions" of these items, but if you can't go to the store and buy them, it's not a problem. Get creative: use any old blankets, pillows, belts, towels or even shoe boxes in your house to assist you! Essentially anything sturdy and comfortable can be used as a prop.

Do you know that a pencil and paper is also a prop? Along with the stretches, meditating, and breathing exercises, this book will ask you to express yourself with your words through writing. At the end of each chapter, there is a writing journal section in which you can reflect on different questions and thoughts. It is important for you to know that your words and thoughts are important. The world wants (and needs) to hear your ideas. It just makes this place better.

You may be wondering how yoga can be done by writing. When you write you are able to get to know yourself better and also be really honest. This allows you to practice Limbs 1 (Yamas) and 2 (Niyamas) and your Throat Chakra. Writing is a form of expression. Your words are important. Keep a journal to let them out! You can share your answers with others or keep them private.

How does yoga bring peace?

Sometime life is happy. Sometimes life is sad. Sometimes we get mad or angry or nervous or scared. Sometimes we have really good days full of fun and laughter. Sometimes we have sad days where we may cry or feel sick. Yoga teaches you how to take care of your body and mind so you can have more happy days than sad, and when you have sad days, yoga teaches you how to get through them a little easier. All of these lessons will help bring you peace.

Remember when we talked about giving? Give everything you learn to your friends! Be a yoga teacher to them, inspiring them to bring peace and health to their body and mind, too. Tell them about the limbs. Everyone can be a yogi, and everyone is a teacher. We all learn from each other. How cool would it be if every teen in the world was peaceful and healthy?

Chapter 2

Yoga for Gratitude

Remember the focus of yoga is to bring peace. As humans, we all have a lot of emotions. Because you are a teen, and your hormones are changing, you have even more emotions. This is totally tough.

Lots of things happen as a teenager. The subjects you learn about in school are different and harder so you learn a lot of stuff. This can be overwhelming. You also meet lots of new friends in school and other activities, which causes you to get closer or move away from your old friends. You really start to understand what it means to have a good friend. These friendships are special. You even may start to have a boyfriend or girlfriend and get to experience first love.

You also get treated more like an adult. You are not a little kid anymore, and this is really cool. You get to think about things like what you want to be and do when you grow up. You get to figure out what hobbies and things you like to do. You start to really define your personality and understand what makes you, you. This is super special.

You also get more freedom. You will learn to drive (if you aren't driving already). You even will get to think about what you will do after high school. You'll get to explore really amazing ideas like: Will you go to college? What will your job be? Who will you become when you grow up?

All of this stuff is awesome. Sometimes, though, it can cause lots of pressure and stress in your mind. Yoga shows that when your mind is stressed, your body is stressed. This means to help de-stress your mind, you need to de-stress your body.

The exercises below are going to teach you how to de-stress your body so you can de-stress your mind and come to that place of bliss we talked about.

When de-stressing your body and mind, it's really important to focus on a positive emotion. For this chapter we are going to focus on being grateful.

You have so much to be grateful for. Do you know how many adults wish they were teenagers again? The time is yours: appreciate it every second!

Teenagers learn so much, change so much, and get to have so much fun, but sometimes, teens forget all that they have and want more. This can cause you to be "bratty" or even spoiled. The opposite can also happen: if you don't have a lot and aren't grateful for the little you do have, this can cause you to be bitter or sad. A lot of times this happens because we look at others and wish we had what they had. I know so many times as a teen I wished I looked like someone else or had a boyfriend like other girls did.

Wanting to be something or someone else, makes you not appreciative of the person you are and the life you are living. There is nothing more important than you, and whatever is happening in your life is perfect (even if it is hard stuff). By me wishing I looked different or had something different than I did, it pulled me away from acknowledging and appreciating the great stuff I did have.

Many teens also like STUFF: having stuff, getting stuff and buying stuff is important for many teenagers. I really thought having a lot of stuff was important and cool when I was a teen. I didn't realize the value of money, and I would constantly ask my parents to buy me things and get upset if I didn't get them. Sometimes when my parents did buy me something and I didn't like it, I would get mad.

Wanting lots of stuff is an immature thought. Stuff really isn't important, although it may seem it. Stuff provides us a false sense of happiness that goes away after a while. Think about when you were a little kid and got a present. At first, it was probably super exciting, but after a while you probably didn't notice it or appreciate it, and after a little more time, you probably never played with it. This is how Christmas was for me when I was a little kid. I would be so happy for a few days, then I'd be bored with all my stuff after a while, and before I knew it, all my once cool, new things were old, and I wanted something else. There was no gratitude here.

This habit has followed me as an adult: I have a closest full of clothes, and I don't wear half of them, yet I always want to go shopping and buy more. This not only wastes money, but causes stress. Wanting things holds us back from appreciating things we do have—important things like our health, body, mind, positivity, nature, love, family and friends. It also gives us a feeling of urgency. We begin to feel anxiety or stress by having or not having stuff, and this pulls us away from being as peaceful as we could be, and being peaceful links directly to being more happy and healthy.

Be so appreciative for everything that happens to you. It will make you a stronger, smarter, and happier adult. Be so appreciative for everything you have. Things are things, and really when you think about them, they aren't that important.

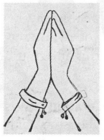

Dylan Age 11

Stretches
Sun Salutations
(*Surya Namaskara*)

Surya means "sun," and Namaskara means "salute." A Sun Salutation is a powerful series of poses that not only stretches and strengthens all parts of your body, but also teaches a valuable lesson about appreciation and honor!

When you do a Sun Salutation, you are honoring and appreciating the "sun." The sun represents two different things. First, the sun represents the actual sun, that big ball of fire in the universe keeping our earth alive. When you move through the poses of the Sun Salutation, you are saying "thank you" to the sun as it is the giver of life (as I'm sure you learned about in Science class).

Arms Over Head Pose, Half-Forward Fold Pose, and **Upward Facing Dog** represent the different states of the sun rising.

Forward Fold, Four Limb Staff Pose, and **Downward Facing Dog** represent the different stages of the sun setting.

Also, when you do a Sun Salutation you are honoring the metaphoric sun that lives within you—your heart! Your heart is the sun of your body: it keeps you alive (just as the sun keeps the Earth alive) and this is something that should be honored.

When you think about life this way, having the coolest shoes or wanting to be someone you're not, seems just silly. You are you, and you are alive under this amazing sun that gives us food and life! How cool is that?

When you do a Sun Salutation you are physically giving your heart a powerful energy boost as each pose helps with moving circulation in the body.

Your beating heart is something to be so grateful for. Think about it; your body is constantly working. Your blood is flowing and your heart is beating. Your heart beats an average of 100,000 times a day. I don't know anyone who would do 100,000 things for me a day, every day. We definitely need to say thank you to our heart.

When you do a Sun Salutation you start with your palms pressed into one another like this:

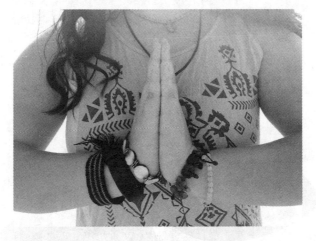

This is called "Namaskara Mudra," which is the name for the hand position that shows you are grateful.

There are various types of Sun Salutations: here is a basic one.

First, stand in **Mountain Pose** with your hands in **Namaskara Mudra**. Then take an **inhale** and raise your hands to **Arms Over Head Pose**. Then take an **exhale** and do a **Forward Fold**. Then take an inhale and do **Half Forward Fold Pose**. Then go to a **Four Limb Staff Pose** on an exhale. Take an inhale and go into **Upward Facing Dog Pose**. Then take an exhale and go into **Downward Facing Dog Pose**. Then come back to a **Forward Fold** and on your inhale go back into **Arms Over Head Pose**. Finally come back to **Mountain Pose**, on an exhale, bringing your hands at **Namaskara Mudra**. Notice the breathing here. Each move has a breath. The breathing is a big part in defining how a Sun Salutation works. The breath, just like the sun, is the giver and sustainer of life.

If you are confused about all these poses, their order, and how to do them, don't worry. The following pages show the poses of a Sun Salutation explained step by step.

Mountain Pose
(*Tadasana*)

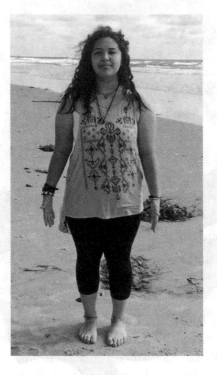

How do I do it?

Stand up tall with your feet flat, firm against the ground. Bring your arms down by your side. Let the palms of your hands face forward.

To improve the pose:

- Lift and spread your toes and lift the balls of your feet and lay them softly down on the ground.

- Tighten your thigh muscles and lift your knee caps.

- Keep your belly relaxed.

- Lift your inner ankles to strengthen the inner arches.

- With your arms along your side, shrug your shoulders up towards your ears and down your back.

- Place your chin parallel to the ground.

- Stand strong and rooted into the ground.

- Breathe easily.

Why should I do it?

By just standing in this pose, you have a chance to feel this body that is yours. Feel your body—how can you not be grateful for your spine and how strong it holds you up? You are so lucky. Appreciate this pose: it feels really good especially because you probably do a lot of sitting in school.

This pose is named "Mountain Pose." When you're standing in this pose, think about a mountain: it gets climbed on, lived on, and rain and snowed on, but it stays super strong. It cannot move. This is you! You are strong like a mountain. Stand tall and don't let any of the problems you face try to bring you down. You do this best by being grateful.

This poses also:

- Stretches your hands, feet, and neck.

- Makes your feet feel really strong.

- Relieves any back aches.

- Firms your belly.

- Strengthens your thighs, knees, and ankles

- Improves your posture (texting and playing on the computer makes it hard for us to have great posture).

- Makes you feel strong (like you're on top of the world!).

Arms Above Head Pose
(*Urdvha Hastasana*)

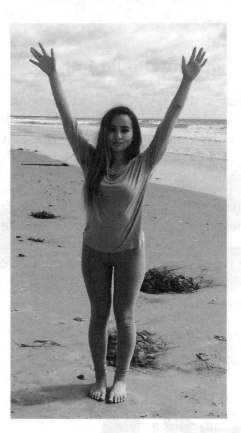

How do I do it?

Standing tall with your feet touching or with a space between them, raise your arms all the way up above your head. Keep your arms straight and have your palms face into one another.

To improve the pose:

- Shrug your shoulders close up by your ears, and then relax your shoulders down keeping your spine nice and strong.

- Lift up your toes, and then place each toe down one by one. Feel your feet pressed really firm on the floor.

- Inhale deeply and feel your ribs and lungs rise up.

- Be sure your upper arms are framing your ears.

- Don't lock your knees. If you need to, bend your knees just a little so your knees don't get stiff.

Why should I do it?

By reaching your arms up high, but staying grounded in your feet, you're able to feel how strong your body is and how long it can stretch. Yoga actually can make you a little taller because you're stretching your body so deeply. Feel how high you can reach your arms over your head. Be grateful for how alive your arms feel in this position; as you are reversing the blood flow in your arms bringing all new, fresh, oxygen-rich blood to your whole body by just doing this pose!

This pose also:

- Makes your leg muscles strong.

- Makes your spine longer (you'll feel taller!).

- Stretches your abs, shoulders and armpits.

- Helps relieve anxiety and nervousness.

- Gives you energy if you're feeling tired.

- Helps you breathe better (this pose is great for people with asthma).

- Helps get rid of any aches in your back.

Forward Fold
(*Uttanasana*)

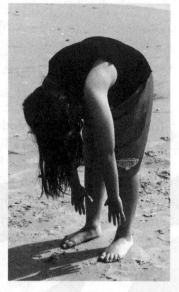

How do I do it?
Bend from your hips, letting your arms hang down resting your hands on your shins, heals, or the floor. The goal is to fold your body in half! You can bend your knees if you need to.

To improve the pose:

- Give in to gravity, allow your entire upper body to just hang.

- Bend your knees and then straighten your legs to make your leg muscles less tense.

- Relax your neck and let your head hang loose.

- Your feet can be together or slightly separated, but press your feet firmly in the ground.

- Use a block to rest your hands if they don't reach the floor.

- Be sure to breathe!

Why should I do it?

By forward folding, you are really allowing gravity to work with you. Your back muscles will feel less tight because of this. Open your eyes in this pose. See the world from a new perspective; let this inspire you in your life right-side up, and then be grateful for this view.

This pose also:

- Strengthens the spine.

- Stretches the hamstrings.

- Relaxes your body.

- Helps your body digest things (this is a really good pose to do after you eat too much!).

Four Limbs Staff Pose
(*Chaturanga Dandasana*)

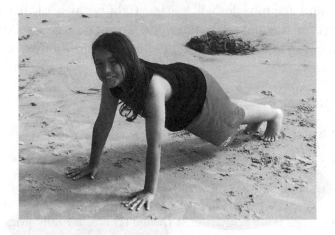

How do I do it?

This pose is just like holding a push up, only your elbows are tucked in (not pointing out). Place your hands on the ground and walk your feet back so you are in a plank position: your spine, shoulders, head and hips are in one long straight line. Hang an inch or two above the ground.

You are on your toes and your heels are super active, pushing as if there was a wall behind you. Your core should feel on fire. Your arms may shake. This pose tests your strength, so you can come down on your knee at any time to take some pressure off your core and arms: still tighten your core and arms, and keep your shoulders, hips, head and spine in that straight, even line.

To improve the pose:

- Keep your hands active: spread your fingers wide and push the earth away from you.

- Keep your elbows bent, tucked close to your body.

- Squeeze in your belly.

- Go to where you feel most comfortably challenged.

Why should I do it?

This pose reminds you that you are strong. It builds your core and arm muscles by giving you lots of strength. Remember this pose whenever you are feeling weak. You are powerful!

This pose also:

- Strengthens your shoulders.

- Builds your arm muscles.

- Makes your wrists strong.

- Makes your abs really toned.

Upward Dog
(*Urdhva Mukha Svanasana*)

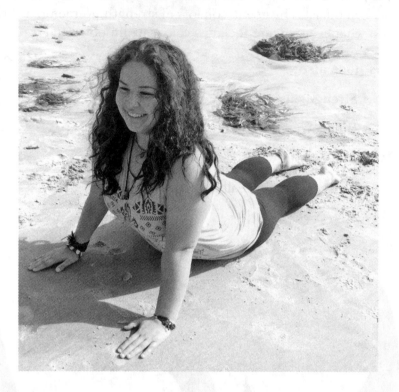

How do I do it?
From Four Limbs Staff Pose, press the top of your feet (the toenail side of the foot) into the ground. Your thighs and hips are lifted off the ground. Your chest is back, and your throat is stretching as you are looking up. Your fingers are spread wide as your hands press into the ground.

To improve the pose:

- Keep your arms straight.

- Keep your shoulders down and away from your ears.

- Try to lift your thighs and knees.

- Open your heart.

- Breathe deeply feeling the air come from your nostrils down to your open chest.

Why should I do it?

This pose teaches the importance of opening your heart. Do you feel all that space you are creating within your chest in this pose? When you open your heart, you allow your life is be filled with more love. That is something to be grateful for and Upward Facing Dog reminds of this.

This pose also:

- Makes your spine stronger.

- Stretches the muscles in your belly.

- Improves your arm strength.

- Stretches your feet (you use your feet constantly and don't even think about it, so this pose is amazing for that).

- Helps keep your metabolism in balance.

Downward Facing Dog
(*Adho Mukha Svanasana*)

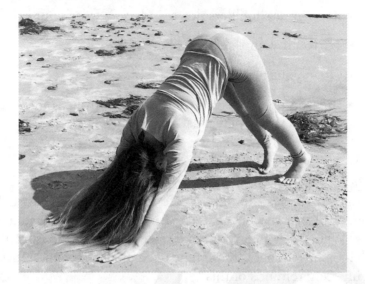

How do I do it?
You are going to make an upside-down V-shape with your body while having your hands and feet on the floor. To do this, come on to all-fours (just like a dog). Lift your hips up high as you straighten both of your legs. Let your head hang (with strength and control) in between your arms.

To improve the pose:

- Spread all ten fingers super wide. Try to make a "J" shape with your index finger and thumb as you really press your hands into the ground.

- The higher you can get your hips, the better. Try bending your knees to lift your hips up higher.

- In this pose you are hanging upside down, so don't forget to breathe or you may become dizzy!

- Ideally your legs should be hip-width distance and your arms should be shoulder-width distance apart from each other.

- Your hands and feet should be 4 to 5 feet away from each other.

- Work on getting your heels flat to the ground.

Why should I do it?

Watch any dog, and they will do this pose at least once a day. Why? It feels really good because it stretches pretty much everything. Just like dogs do, give your body a full stretch every day, and send gratitude for this good feeling.

This pose also:

- Loosens tight muscles in the back of your legs.

- Makes your shoulders and neck feel really good.

- Gives you more energy because you are hanging upside down (so your blood flow is being flipped: this is really cool because it helps bring more oxygen to your blood).

- Makes your arms really strong.

- Helps keep your spine long and tension-free.

Tips for Sun Salutations

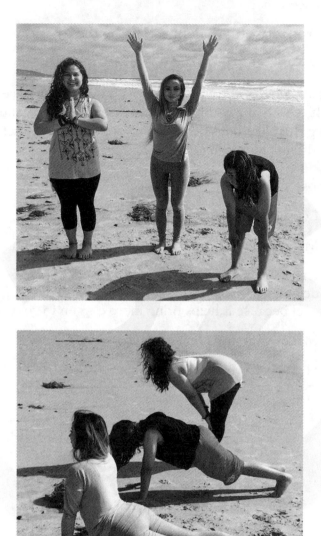

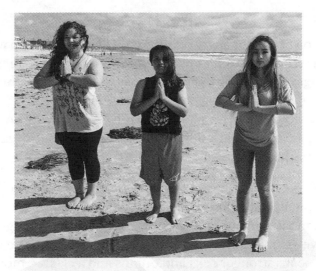

You can do all of these poses by themselves, or you can do them together as a Sun Salutation. If you do them as a Sun Salutation just remember:

- Take one breath for each movement.

- Send gratitude for the sun and your sun every time you do the series of poses.

- Do as many as your heart (your sun!) desires.

- Always take a break if you get tired.

- There are many versions of Sun Salutations, and this is just one. Make up your own. Be grateful in each movement!

Breathing

When you're tired or angry or busy, your lungs never stop working for you. When you don't feel like you want to do anything, your diaphragm (the muscle that is responsible for your breathing) still keeps moving. We inhale and exhale all day, every day: we need to or we would die. The act of breathing is mainly subconscious (meaning we do it naturally without thinking), but yoga allows us to breathe consciously.

Breathing consciously not only helps us take fuller breaths in the moment, but it also helps us build our diaphragm muscle so we can take fuller breathes subconsciously in our regular life when we are not doing yoga. Fuller breaths mean more oxygen which means stronger cells and organs and a clearer, more calm mind. This is something to be thankful for!

At least once a day, stop and take a few minutes to send gratitude to your breath, lungs and diaphragm. You can do this when you wake up, before you go to bed, when you are waiting in line at lunch…whenever you feel like it.

Here's one way to connect with your lungs:

- Place your right hand over your right lung.

- Place your left hand over your left lung.

- Close your eyes and feel your hands move up and down as you inhale and exhale.

- Notice the rhythm of your breath. Smile at this movement and thank your lungs.

- Then, when you're ready, start to take deeper and slower inhales and exhales.

- Take your time. Really feel your entire respiratory system (the organs and structures in your body responsible for your breathing) as they do their job.

- Send a big thank you to this system!

Meditation

Something that will help you when you meditate is to have a "mantra." Mantra is Sanskrit for "mind tool." It is a word or phrase that helps you focus and calm your mind. To keep your focus on gratitude, you can use a mantra in your meditation.

Here's how:

- Get in a comfortable position. Maybe you sit or lay down. It doesn't matter. Just get comfortable.

- Close your eyes and start to focus inward not letting the outside world distract you (this is Pratyahara: this means to try your best not to let any of the natural sounds, smells, sights, etc. pull your mind away from what you are doing, which is meditating).

- Take a deep inhale. As you inhale, say to yourself the word: *"Thank."*

- Take a deep exhale. As you exhale, say to yourself the word: *"You."*

- *"Thank you"* will be your mantra.

- Try to meditate in this way for at least five minutes. The longer you can stay focused the better. But, even one minute of meditation a day will make your body and mind stronger than it was before.

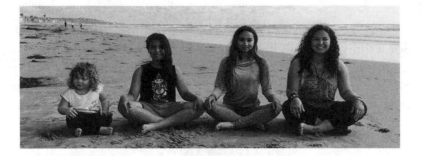

Writing

Do you know what the best part about gratitude is? It's like a magnet. The more grateful and appreciative you are, the more you get to be grateful for.

Every night before you go to bed make a quick gratitude list: keep a journal and call it your "Thank You Book." Write down everything that happened to you that day that you are grateful for.

Look back at this book when you are feeling sad, as it will make you feel better. Look at this book when you are happy too: notice how your lists get longer and longer each day as you attract more things in your life to be thankful for.

Chapter 3

Yoga for Focus

You must have a lot of stuff going on in that head of yours, huh? Don't worry: I have a lot of stuff going on in my head too.

When I was a teen, I thought there was something wrong with me for thinking so much. I definitely felt I was a freak with too many ideas going on in my head. I would think about everything. I'd get sad or happy thinking about stuff that already happened. I'd get nervous or excited thinking about stuff that was going to happen. I became super worried thinking about stuff that could happen. Sometimes I even got a headache from all of those thoughts.

I remember sitting in my math class (I hated math: it was so hard for me! But, on a side note: I'm a full time yoga teacher, and I use math every day of my life. Sure, I'm not graphing integers, but all of the concepts I learned in all of my math classes help me as an adult—for real.) Anyway, as I'd sit in math class and draw in my notebook or stare out the window, I'd think lots and lots of thoughts. If I was in high school today, I'd probably get diagnosed with ADD. ADD did not really exist 17 years ago. (If you pay attention in math, you can figure out how old I am: **x=my age, age of a freshman in high school + 17=x**).

Today, it seems everyone's talking about ADD, and everyone is giving their kids pills to stop them from thinking so much. I read a statistic the other day that said that 2 million American teens have ADD. So, if you have been diagnosed with ADD, don't worry, 1, 999,999 teens have been too. (See, I just used math.)

The thing is, everyone thinks a lot. Every single person. Thinking a lot or being in your head is human. It is not wrong or a bad thing. It's actually pretty amazing how complex our brain is and how it has the ability to think in many different ways from many different angles.

The problem with thinking a lot happens when we don't live in the present moment because we are living in our head. This is what happened to me. I kept thinking and thinking and thinking. This forced me to not pay attention. My friends would always joke about how clumsy I was: I'd always trip over things because I wasn't paying attention. I was thinking too much in my head. I'd also make lots of mistakes, and I'd forget things too.

My favorite thing to think about as a teen was the future. I wanted to know who I was going to marry and what I was going to be when I grew up. I wondered what college I'd get into and where I would live. I fantasized about what my job would be and what my kids would look like. All this time in my head thinking about what could happened, made me miss out on what was happening in front of me.

The funny thing is: everything I thought about never happened. I swore I was going to marry my high school boyfriend, Mike Hickman, be an elementary school teacher and have two kids living in New Jersey. Mikey and I would have two houses: one in the town we went to high school in and one by the beach. We'd afford these houses because he'd be a really rich computer guy (computers were just getting popular then). I thought he was really good at computers because we always chatted on AOL IM (the first form of Social Media) and he would send me things like this: **:)** or **<3** . I definitely would have a cat because I hated dogs. Oh, and all of this stuff would happen by the time I was 25 years old.

Guess where I am right now? If you did the math, you know my age, and even though I may seem ancient since I lived in a time before the internet existed, I'm about six years older than 25. Mikey and I broke up about 14 years ago. I am not married, and I don't have any kids. I live in San Diego, paying for my own beach-front apartment all by myself. My job is a yoga teacher (I had no idea what yoga was when I was in high school). I write books and teach people how to use yoga to calm their life. I also have two, little, barking dogs. I would have never thought this would be my life when I was in high school.

If you would have told "high school Shawna" any of this, she would have thought "Adult Shawna" was such a loser. She'd be confused about how and why she wasn't married, and she definitely wouldn't understand why she wasn't still with Mikey. Now "Adult Shawna" thinks "High School Shawna" was just a cute, daydreamer.

I'm telling you all of this because, most likely, you think a lot too. Our thoughts like to hang out in the past (I still remember Mikey's AOL screen name) or in the future (I still wonder who I'm going to marry), but all of these thoughts about the past and future, rob us of the present moment. Most likely, if I wasn't fantasizing about what my life would be like after high school, and I would have paid better attention in high school, I probably would have done better in math.

As a teen, I know you have a lot on your mind. I also know you have a lot of pressures, and sometimes this can cause you to over-focus. Your grades are important, your extra-curricular activities and any sports you play are important; if you have a job, that's important too. You also have friends, family, and maybe a boyfriend or girlfriend to pay attention to, also. You have a lot to focus on and focusing on the present moment can be overwhelming.

Basically, when we aren't focused, two things can happen: first, we can be way so much in our head that we don't pay attention to what is happening and we miss lots of stuff. Second, we can become obsessive. So much so that we start to notice small things, and these things can start to drive us crazy, like not putting things in their "right spot." This obsessive compulsive behavior starts as a teenager (or younger) and follows way into adulthood. I know lots of adults who are known as "clean freaks" or something else because they are so fixated on controlling the small details, they lose focus of the purpose of life or being present.

Yoga teaches us how to live in the present moment and be focused and peaceful in each moment. This is really important for teens to understand because the reality of life is all that matters is this very second. You can't change the past and you can't control the future. All you can do is be the best you, right here, right now.

The exercises below are going to inspire you to be present. They will teach you how to control your thoughts, so you can be focused on the moment. It's important to set goals for the future and be grateful for your past, but you want to be able to do so without getting lost in your thoughts.

Stretches: Standing Poses

Standing Poses teach you to be in the here and now. In all of these poses, by pressing your feet firmly into the ground, you are reminded of the present moment. Your feet allow you to feel strong, while the rest of your body continues to grow and stretch. In these poses, your focus is so important. You must be sure you are doing the pose correctly so you can get the greatest benefit out of it.

Standing poses are the most powerful when you hold them for a set amount of time. Focusing on your breath and how your body feels in these poses will allow you to develop stronger body awareness. From this awareness, you will be able to be more in your body and less in your head in your everyday life.

Extended Triangle Pose
(*Utthita Trikonasana*)

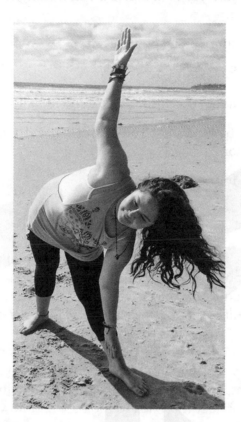

How do I do it?

Stand in Mountain pose and then separate your legs as far as you comfortably can (usually this is about 3 to 4 feet away from each other). Have your front foot facing straight forward, and your back foot facing horizontally (making about a ninety-degree angle). Your heels should be in a line with each other (you could literally draw a perfectly straight line from your front heel to your back heel). Reach both of your arms really far out to the sides. Then inch forward, allowing your hand to come down wherever it comfortably falls. Reach your top arm up, opening your chest and shoulders, keeping your shoulders in line with one another. Be sure to do this pose on both sides of your body!

To improve the pose:

- Make sure your shoulders are in a straight line with one another.

- Make sure your hips are even.

- Don't lock your knees.

- Look up at your upwardly extended hand.

- Use a block to rest your lower hand if you can't reach the floor.

- Don't forget to breathe.

Why should I do it?

Do you know notice all the triangles you are making with your body in this pose? You are making 3 triangles: one triangle with your arms, another with your legs, and a last triangle with your entire body. All of the yoga poses have a deep, symbolic meaning behind them. Triangle Pose honors the special number three. As you are standing strong and focusing on this pose, use this pose to help you to remember to honor all the "3's" in your life: like your past, present, and future, and your mind, body, and soul. Then connect this back to the here and now.

This pose also:

- Strengthens your thighs, knees, and ankles.

- Stretches your hips, groins, hamstrings, calves, shoulders, chest, and spine.

- Brings health to all the organs related to digestion (allowing you to digest foods and thoughts better).

- Helps release neck and back pain (maybe caused from too much texting or typing).

- Helps relieve stress.

Chair Pose
(*Utkatasana*)

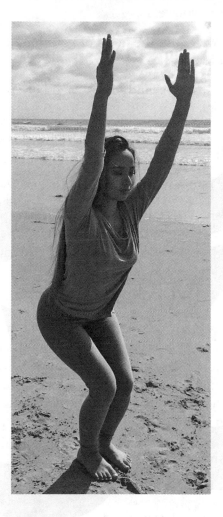

How do I do it?

Chair Pose is sort of like a half squat. From Mountain Pose, with your feet together, bend your knees and raise your arms overhead. Squeeze your legs together as you bend. You are in a slight squat and should feel like you are sitting in a tiny, imaginary chair that is right behind you.

To improve the pose:

- Keep your chest lifted, but bring your shoulders down away from your ears.

- Put the weight in the heels of your feet: lift your toes so you can feel this.

- Press your thighs and knees together. Your legs should be parallel.

- Look down to make sure you can see your toes. If you can't, sit back further on your "chair."

- Breathe into anywhere your body feels tight.

- If your shoulders are tight or it hurts to put your hands up above your head, bring your arms straight out in front of you.

Why should I do it?

Chair Pose is also known as "Fierce Pose." Old Indian mythology believes that warriors got their strength from their muscles. This poses draws a lot of strength from the muscles within the body, especially the thighs. Focus on this fierceness and strength when in this pose. Then use this in your life when you feel weak, lost in your thoughts, or removed from the present moment.

This pose also:

- Teaches balance.

- Helps you to stay focused.

- Builds your endurance.

- Makes your thighs really strong.

Warrior 1
(*Virabhadrasana 1*)

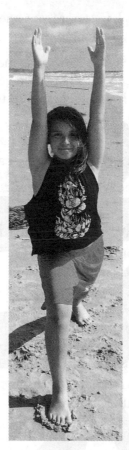

How do I do it?
Standing in Mountain Pose, bring one foot back about 4 to 5 feet. If you drew a line from your front heel to your back heel, they would intersect each other (this is referred to as "heel-to-heel alignment"). Then bring your hands on your hips. Be sure your hips stay facing forward. Bend into your front knee. Move your back foot out to whatever angle you need to get your hips facing forward. You can even lift your heel up, but the goal is to get your back foot flat on the ground facing a 45 degree angle. Reach your arms straight overhead, your pinkies facing one another. Breathe. Be focused and strong. You are a warrior! Be sure to do this pose on both sides of your body!

To improve the pose:

- Press your feet really firmly into the floor.

- Try your best to have your front knee bent to a 90 degree angle (Look at all of the math we are using!)

- Having your hips face forward is the most important part of this pose. Keep your hands on your hips to keep them facing forward if you feel one hip is moving back.

- If you can, press your palms together over your head. Keep your arms nice and straight and bring your shoulders down and back (away from your ears).

- Squeeze your belly in: keep your core strong!

Why should I do it?

There are three warrior poses in yoga. These poses represent the physical and symbolic energy of a warrior in different phases of battle. These poses make your body feel really strong in the muscles of your legs which symbolizes vitality and power. Also, in all of the warrior poses, your chest is open: this is a reminder to fight with focused peace and love. True warriors stand up for what is right; being strong through love, not violence. They need to be focused, in the present moment, so they can stand up strong and not make a mistake.

In Warrior 1, the body is facing forward. This is a reminder to face our problems in a focused way, that is head on. Be strong and compassionate in confrontations, always being a warrior for peace

This pose also:

- Builds stamina.

- Builds endurance (which makes you able to last longer for study sessions or classes and late-night practices).

- Improves flexibility.

- Makes the legs, feet and thighs stronger.

- Helps the knees and hips be steady and strong.

Warrior 2
(*Virabhadrasana 2*)

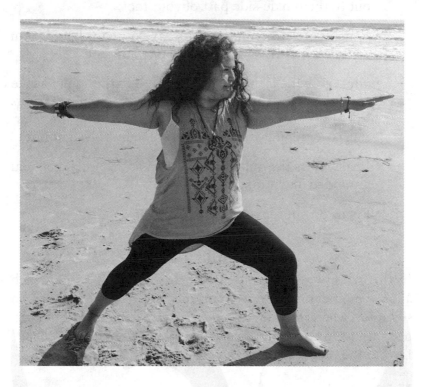

How do I do it?

Standing in Mountain Pose, bring one foot back about 4 to 5 feet. It differs from Warrior I in that, if you drew a line from your front heel to your back foot, it would intersect at the arch of your foot (this is referred to as "heel-to-arch alignment"). Your back foot should be at a 90 degree angle. Then bring your hands on your hips. Be sure your hips stay facing the direction the back toes are pointing. Keep your hips in this even direction and bend in the front knee to a 90 degree angle. Spread your arms really wide out to your side. Turn your head and look over the fingers of the arm out in front of you. Focus here. Breathe and stay strong. Be sure to do this pose on both sides of your body.

To improve the pose:

- To get a deep stretch along the thigh, press the front knee out to the pinkie-side part of your foot.

- Reach your arms out as wide as you can: keep them completely even and parallel to one another.

- Your tail-bone is the bone at the base of the spine. Make sure it is not sticking out in this pose. Often times teachers will say "Tuck your tail-bone." This is what they are referring to (bringing your hips and spine in a straight line).

- Really press the outer edge of the back foot to keep you grounded and strong.

- Focus on your breathing.

Why should I do it?

In this second Warrior pose, your arms are out wide, which allows your heart to be open. This teaches that when you are in situations where you may need to stand up for what is right; you need to do so strong and peaceful, focused on an open heart. Love is the only way to win a battle.

This pose also:

- Tones your legs.

- Encourages deep focus.

- Builds your endurance in your muscles.

- Stretches your hips.

- Improves your posture.

- Makes your feet strong.

- Physically and emotionally opens your heart.

Extended Wide Leg Bend
(*Prasarita Padottanasana*)

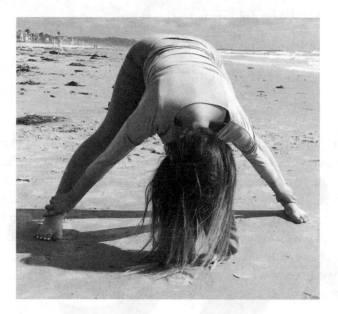

How do I do it?

From Mountain Pose, walk your legs out as wide as you can. Put your hands on your hips, and then forward fold. Rest your hands wherever they comfortably fall. Look at the world through your legs upside down.

To improve the pose:

- Be sure to keep your knees, feet, hips, and chest forward.

- Your feet should be parallel to one another.

- Press your feet firmly into the ground.

- Bend your knees a little if the muscles in the back of your legs are tight.

- Breathe (sometimes you forget when you are hanging upside down).

- Bend your elbows, and firmly press your hands to the floor directly below you.

Try different hand placements for different stretches:

- Bring your hands to your hips.

- Bring your forearms to the floor.

- Interlace your hands behind your back.

- Reach for your big toes.

Why should I do it?

It is important to be focused from all angles of your life, Whether you need to focus your emotions or thoughts when talking to someone to express yourself your clearest, or you need to focus to do the task at hand to the best of your ability, focusing is a practice that reminds you to be in the present moment only (not the past or the future). When you're hanging upside down in this pose, remind yourself that no matter what you're doing, what you see or where your head is, being focused will give you the best results!

This pose also:

- Makes your feet and legs stable (so you will be less likely to fall or be a clumsy person; this will also make your more attentive when you are doing sports and other physical activities!)

- Stretches your shoulders

- Gives your energy

- Recharges your mind (this is really helpful in getting you focused or if you are focusing too much!)

Extended Side Angle Stretch
(*Utthita Parsvakonasana*)

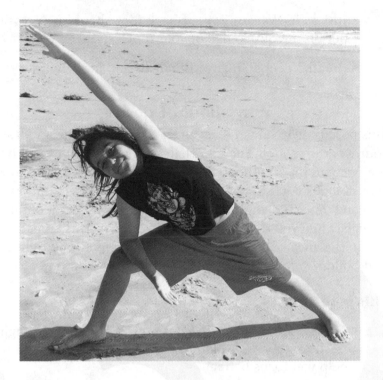

How do I do it?

It is easiest to come to this pose from Warrior 2. Once you're in Warrior 2, reach your arms and body forward a few inches, then bend your elbow and rest it on your thigh. Press your shoulders back and reach your back arm up. Keep your shoulders and hips in line with one another.

To improve the pose:

- You can look up to your extended hand.

- You can bring your hand down to the ground or a block, instead of resting on your thigh. When you make this adjustment, be sure to keep the chest open and shoulders and hip in a line.

Your front knee should be kept bent at a 90 degree angle:

- don't let your knees go so far out you can't see your toes.

- Just as in Warrior 2, your back foot should be pressing out on the outer edge of your foot.

- Breathe deeply to give your arms and legs energy.

Why should I do it?

This pose is deep lunge. A teenager's job is to study and learn: your work is school! The knowledge school provides will help prepare you for adulthood and all the jobs you will do and responsibilities you will have in your adult life. It is so important to spend time studying and focusing on learning. A lot of times, though, when you study, you are sitting down. This lunge is the counterbalance of all that sitting. It will help all the tightness that builds up from being seated throughout your day.

This pose also:

- Gives you energy as it helps your circulation (bringing fresh, oxygen-rich blood flow to your body, which will help you focus better).

- Stretches the side of your body, including the little muscles along the rib cage.

- Helps make your chest and shoulders strong.

- Relieves any back, thigh, and hip tightness caused by sitting.

Pyramid Pose
(*Parsvottanasana*)

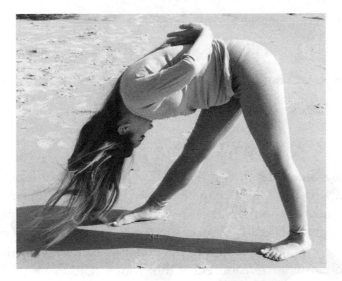

How do I do it?

Standing in Mountain Pose, bring one leg back about 3 to 4 feet. The separation in your legs is shorter than when it is in the Warrior poses. Put your hands on your hips and have your hips facing forward. Try to have both of your feet facing forward. If you can't do this, don't worry. You can move your back foot to the angle you need to keep your hips in a straight line. Keep your front leg straight and start to bend forward over the leg. Allow your hands to stay at your hips as you bend forward. Breathe here and focus on releasing all of the tension in your body. Be sure to do this pose on both sides of your body.

To improve the pose:

• Always be sure your hips are facing forward.

You can make this pose more difficult by adjusting your hand placement

• You can place your hands on the ground

- You can place your hands behind your back— try to grab for opposite elbows or press your palms together behind your back for Reversed Namaste Mudra.

- Relax your neck.

- Have your ribs be parallel with the floor.

- Relax your belly.

- Focus on your breathing.

Why should I do it?

Intense Side Stretch is intense! It releases a lot of tension in your body. This tension can be caused by over-focusing. Maybe you study for hours and hours without standing up, moving your body and taking a break. Maybe an hour goes by as you're playing on your phone or watching television. Sitting in a desk in school can cause tension. All of this brings tightness to the body.

It's also important to be sure to keep physical and mental balance in your body. What this means is don't focus too much in your head without giving focus to your body too. If you are thinking and thinking about something (which can often make you worried, sad, or angry), your muscles are going to get tight from the worry, sadness or anger in your body.

Wherever your focus is, be sure to bring it back to your physical health. This pose stretches from the back of your heels all the way up your neck, releasing tension throughout your entire back of your body.

This pose also:

- Stretches your hips.

- Helps relieve muscle pain.

- Helps tightness in your neck.

- If you do Reversed Namaste Mudra, you'll get a nice stretch in your elbows and wrists.

Breathing

Breathing is something done, most of the time, without focus. Let's change that!

Here's how:

- Get comfortable.

- Bring your focus to your breathing.

- Bring your hand to the right side of your lung (on your right side of your chest).

- Bring your left hand to the left side of your lung (on your left side of your chest).

- Inhale really deep through your nose.

- Focus on the air traveling all the way down your throat into your chest. Feel both of your hands (and your lungs) raise up.

- Really focus on your lungs — picture them as balloons and try to fill them up with as much air as you can.

- When you can't fill up your lungs anymore, exhale all of the air of your chest. Picture your lungs now as deflating balloons. Take notice as to where the air comes out!

- Now start to count your breaths: breathe in for 2 counts, and then breathe out for two counts.

- Repeat these steps trying your hardest to focus on how you breathe and for how long (increase the number of breaths whenever you want)!

Meditating

Meditation is all about focus. In fact, the entire point of meditation is to focus on the present moment and nothing else. This may same easy, but it can be difficult. By meditating for just a little every day, it will get easier. Your level of focus in your everyday life will improve too. This is because meditation trains your brain to be aware.

A really great way to learn how to focus when meditating is using a meditation strategy called "Yoga Nidra." Yoda Nidra is a type a meditation where you calm your mind, staying focused on the present moment, by paying attention to each of your specific body parts one moment at a time. A person guides you through this. This makes Yoga Nidra a form of guided meditation.

Guided meditation is different from just sitting down and trying your best to meditate because there is a teacher telling you exactly how to meditate. You can listen to a guided meditation online or by using a music app on your phone. You can also have someone read these directions to you. Remember when we talked about giving and receiving? Pair up with some friends and take turns guiding each other through Yoga Nidra. You will all feel really focused. This is especially good to do before a test, game, or job that you have a lot of pressure to do well in or on.

Yoga Nidra can be done really slow or faster. It can take anywhere from 5 minutes to 60 minutes. It just depends on how fast or slow the person guiding you talks.

Here's a sample of Yoga Nidra:

Remember, you can use any words that suit you, just focus on relaxing each part of the body. You can start on the right or left side of your body and at the top or bottom of your body. It doesn't matter. Just allow the intention to be to focus.

- Lay down in a comfortable position.

- Close your eyes.

- Bring your attention to your entire body. Allow your focus to be on nothing else but your body.

- Then shift your attention to your left foot. Think only about your left foot. Then focus on the left big toe. Relax this toe. Focus on the second toe. Relax this toe. Focus on the third toe. Relax this toe. Focus on the fourth toe. Relax this toe. Focus on the pinky toe. Relax this toe. Relax all of your toes; relax even your toenails.

- Then shift your attention up past your toe-line to the top of your foot.

- Relax this area. Relax all the bones on the top of the left foot.

- Continue to bring your awareness to your left ankle. Focus on relaxing this joint.

- Bring your attention to the heel of your foot. Relax this part of your body.

- Continue to focus on your left foot, relaxing the arch of the left foot.

- Then focus on the ball of the left foot. Relax it completely.

- Shift your attention back up your relaxed, left foot.

- Focus on your ankle.

- Focus on your shin.

- Focus on your knee.

- Focus on your thigh.

- Focus on your left hip.

- Then bring your focus on the back of your leg.

- Focus on the back of the thigh.

- Focus on the back of the knee and the little crease made where your knee bends.

- Focus on your calf and all of muscles on the lower part of your left leg.

- Bring your attention back to your left ankle and then to your left foot.

- Focus on relaxing your entire left leg from the toes to the hip.

- Then shift your attention to your right side.

- Think only about your right foot. Then focus on the right big toe. Relax this toe. Focus on the second toe. Relax this toe. Focus on the third toe. Relax this toe. Focus on the fourth toe. Relax this toe. Focus on the pinky toe. Relax this toe. Relax all of your toes; relax even your toenails.

- Then shift your attention up past your toe-line to the top of your foot. Relax this area. Relax all the bones on the top of the right foot.

- Continue to bring your awareness to your right ankle. Focus on relaxing this joint.

- Bring your attention to the heel of your right foot. Relax this part of your body.

- Continue to focus on your right foot, relaxing the arch of the right foot.

- Then focus on the ball of the right foot. Relax it completely.

- Shift your attention back up your relaxed, right foot.

- Focus on your ankle.

- Focus on your shin.

- Focus on your knee.

- Focus on your thigh.

- Focus on your right hip.

- Then bring your focus on the back of your leg.

- Focus on the back of the thigh.

- Focus on the back of the knee and the little crease made where your knee bends.

- Focus on your calf and all of muscles on the lower part of your right leg.

- Bring your attention back to your right ankle and then to your right foot.

- Focus on relaxing your entire right leg from the toes to the hip.

- Then shift your attention to your pelvis region. Focus on relaxing all of the organs here.

- Relax your belly.

- Relax your chest.

- Relax your heart.

- Then bring your focus on your spine, all the way down to your tail-bone—the bottom of your spine.

- Bring your attention up your spine to each vertebrae.

- Then shift your attention to your shoulder blades.

- Focus on your shoulders.

- Shift focus to your left shoulder.

- Focus on the muscles on the top of your left arm on the front side. Then the backside of your upper left arm.

- Bring your attention to your elbow.

- Focus on the left forearm.

- Focus on the left wrist.

- Focus on the top of the left hand.

- Focus on the thumb. Focus on its fingernail.

- Focus on the index finger. Focus on its fingernail.

- Focus on the middle finger. Focus on its fingernail.

- Focus on the ring finger. Focus on its fingernail.

- Focus on the pinky finger. Focus on its fingernail.

- Focus on the back of the left palm.

- Then shift your focus all the way up your left arm, from your fingers to your shoulder.

- Shift focus across your chest to your right shoulder.

- Focus on the muscles on the top of your left arm on the front side. Then the backside of your upper right arm.

- Bring your attention to your elbow.

- Focus on the right forearm.

- Focus on the right wrist.

- Focus on the top of the right hand.

- Focus on the thumb. Focus on its fingernail.

- Focus on the index finger. Focus on its fingernail.

- Focus on the middle finger. Focus on its fingernail.

- Focus on the ring finger. Focus on its fingernail.

- Focus on the pinky finger. Focus on its fingernail.

- Focus on the back of the right palm.

- Then shift your focus all the way up your right arm, from your fingers to your shoulder.

- Shift focus across your chest to your neck.

- Focus on your throat.

- Focus on your chin.

- Focus on your lips.

- Focus on your mouth: your teeth, tongue, and gums.

- Focus on your left cheek.

- Focus on your right cheek.

- Focus on your nose. Pay attention to your left nostril. Then your right nostril.

- Focus your attention to your left eye.

- Focus on your left eyelid.

- Focus on your left eyelashes.

- Focus on your left eyebrow.

- Focus on the space between both of your eyebrows.

- Focus your attention to your right eye.

- Focus on your right eyelid.

- Focus on your right eyelashes.

- Focus on your right eyebrow.

- Focus on your left ear.

- Focus on your right ear.

- Focus on your forehead.

- Focus on your head.

- Focus on your hair.

- Focus on your brain.

- Focus on your thoughts. Let them be clear.

- Then scan your body: focusing on every part of it from your toes to the top of your head.

- Breathe in deep focusing on sending air to each part of your body.

- Focus here on this for as long as you can, and then only when you are ready, focus your attention slowly back to the world and sit up using this focus to guide you the rest of your day.

Writing

Writing keeps your thoughts organized, and through this organization, you will be more a focused.

Meditative Writing AUMwork 1:
Use writing when you feel overwhelmed, and can't get ahold of your thoughts. Just write your thoughts down...let them all out. This will allow you to be more clear-minded and get back to the present moment.

Tip: This is a really good thing to do if you feel like you can't concentrate on whatever you are doing (for example, studying). Take a break. Write down all your thoughts. Then come back clear-minded and focused.

Meditative Writing AUMwork 2:
If you ever feel like you have too much stuff to do or you feel forgetful, make a to-do list. Write down what you have to do, then cross it off when you complete the task. This really works in keeping you focused and aware of everything you need to do.

Meditative Writing AUMwork 3:
To learn more about yourself and why you may have trouble focusing, answer the following questions. Don't spend too much time thinking about the answers; just write from your heart.

Tip: Answer one question at a time, as opposed to reading all the questions at once. This will help you stay focused on one question at a time.

- What are you doing right now?

- What do you think about a lot? Why do you think about it?

- What are you missing when you are thinking too much?

- What was a mistake you made one time? Why do you think you made it?

- What was a time you did really good at something? Why do you feel you did so well?

Read back your answer to the first question: what are you doing right now? If you didn't answer "Answering this question," then you aren't totally focused in the present moment. Tricked ya!

Chapter 4

Yoga for Anger

Anger is a tough emotion. It can come on quickly and turn us into someone we are not. Anger causes us to be mean and sometimes violent. This causes a lot of damage to ourselves and others.

When I was in middle and high school, it seems there was a lot of anger around. Boys and girls would get into fist fights. They would punch each other and call each other names over the smallest things, like what sneakers they were wearing!

I never got in a fist fight, but I remember whenever there was a fist fight, all of the other teens would get excited and run over to watch! Deep down I hated watching fights. It scared me.

Aside from seeing other kids fight, I would see my parents fight. They got divorced when I was 17, but before that there was yelling in my house. Sometimes they would scream really loud and say the meanest things to each other, a lot of times it would be over something small, like food.

I'm not a really angry person, but every person has anger. It's a human emotion. Anger made me feel uncomfortable, but I saw it a lot, so I guess a part of me thought it was normal, so I remember getting mad a lot as a teen and not expressing it correctly.

One time in high school, one of my "friends" stole my boyfriend! One day, Nick was going out with me. The next day, he was making out with Nadine at a party. That made me so mad. First, I kept in this anger, then I started talking about Nick and Nadine in a bad way to everyone, and then, finally, I just erupted. When I saw Nadine at school, I told her off. I yelled at her in front of everyone! My heart was beating so fast and my voice was so loud. I was really, really mean.

The thing is: this didn't change the situation, all it did was get me worked up and make my body and mind feel worse. I was already mad, and I didn't need to physically and mentally feel bad too.

People will be people, and they may do not nice or dishonest things to you. It's ok to get mad at that. We can't control others, and we can't control how we feel. However, we can control what we do with our emotions and how we express them. Yoga helps with this. It reminds us to be healthy: to take care of our body and mind so a negative situation doesn't get more negative. I totally wish I had yoga as a teen.

Your body is really smart: the cells in your body literally remember anger (it's stored as tension and pain). My body felt that anger and remembered it much more than Nick or Nadine did. Looking back, I know all that negatively expressed anger was a waste of energy. There's nothing more important than your own physical and mental health.

As an adult, people still do dishonest and mean things to me from time to time. However, yoga has taught me to let go. I don't yell at people or hold in anger waiting to erupt. I don't talk about people or say bad things about others. Many adults do though.

There is a lot of anger and hatred in the world. There are adults who fight, do violent things, and yell at others. There are over two million adults in jail currently, and most of them are there because of misused anger.

It seems crazy to think that something kids do, adults do too. Adults shouldn't have a problem with anger, they are adults, right? This isn't true. I think this is because no one taught these adults, when they were young adults, how to appropriately handle the anger within them.

The best way to deal with anger is to acknowledge the emotion and then release it and move on living in the present moment, free from tension. Most people use anger as a mask to their feelings. When my parents yelled at each other about food or my peers punched each other in the face over sneakers, they weren't really mad at each other, the food, or the sneakers. They were mad at themselves for some reason (even if they are not conscious of it). As a teen, realize we all go through this—and being honest with our emotions is the only healthy way to deal with them.

Anger is a cycle: when a child doesn't learn how to deal with anger, they become a teen that doesn't know how to deal with anger; they then become an adult who doesn't know how to deal with anger. Adults are role models, so when children and teens see angry adults, they learn that it is ok to use anger incorrectly. Then there is a whole cycle of anger. Make the cycle stop like I did. Learn how to control your anger now, so you become a peaceful, accepting adult who future generations can model after.

Bullies

Let's talk about bullies. First of all, bullies and bullying are a big problem, and the problem is only getting worse now that there is such a thing as cyber bullying. By definition, a bully is someone who picks on another. Realistically, a bully is a person who doesn't know how to properly deal with his or her anger.

Bullying people is the easy way out: it's super easy to be mean to another person as opposed to dealing with the anger that is inside of them. Most people are bullies because they have a lot of negative emotions within them that they don't know how to handle properly. Instead of doing hard work (which is being honest with yourself and figuring out what these negative emotions are, why they happen, and how to make them go away) people turn into bullies, fueled by the anger deep inside of them. They want to make others feel bad because deep down they feel bad too.

If you are a bully, it's ok. The past is the past. Make a change today. Don't be afraid to do hard work and figure out why you act this way. Bullies are not cool (and never were). Bullies think they are cool because they are fooling themselves. They are not being honest with themselves. There is something deep down inside making them mad. This is normal because we all feel this way from time to time, but it is not ok to make others feel bad because you feel bad. Nothing good will ever come from this. Adult bullies are very unhappy people who don't have much love in their life (even if they fool themselves thinking that they do). No one should live this way.

If you are getting bullied, please don't take it personal. Whoever is bullying you has a lot of anger inside of them. Most likely they are bullying you because they see that you aren't an angry person. Although a bully will never admit this, they pick on you because deep down, they want their emotions to be just like yours. They are jealous that you know how to deal with your anger.

If you are getting bullied, be sure to tell an adult. If you don't feel comfortable with any of the adults in your life, find someone nearby that you can talk to about this. You need someone close to help you: ask a teacher or friend's parent. Of course, you can always email me and talk to me about it too (info@YogaWithShawna.com), but remember people nearby will be able to help you immediately and that's what you need to do.

Most important, remember that bullies do not speak truth: *they speak from a place of fear.*

Anger is a dangerous emotion: it makes people into someone they really aren't. If you are reading this book, I may not know you personally, but I do know all people — no matter what age they are — when they are free from negative emotions, are great people, so I feel confident saying that you are great simply because you are reading a book teaching you how to be free from negative emotions. The stretches, breathing exercises, meditation tips, and writing exercises below will help you stay great (or make you even more great!) so you can deal with negative emotions properly when they come into your life. They will also help you be a good role model for all the angry bullies out in the world.

Stretches: Twists

There is a physical component to anger. Anger happens when we can't let go of something. This tension stays energetically in the organs of the body that are responsible for letting go of the toxins in our body (like our liver).

Twists literally help squeeze all that negative anger out of you.

Think about the organs you are positively affecting when you twist. You are helping move all of that anger and stuck toxins out.

Also, anger happens when you are closed minded and only see and understand things from your point of view. When you twist your body, you literally see things from a different perspective. This change of view inspires peace and open-mindedness. Whenever I'm mad, I do a few twists. It helps me push away all that negative energy and come back focused and clear.

Revolving Triangle Pose
(*Parivrtta Trikonasana*)

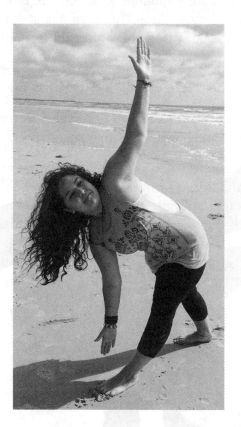

How do I do it?

Standing in Mountain Pose, extend your legs as far as comfortably possible (preferably about 3 to 4 feet) keeping your right foot straight to the front of the mat (facing forward) and your back foot pointing out about 10 to 15 degrees (do whatever feels comfortable for your body). From here, spread your arms out to your sides completely parallel. Inch your body forward, and then lower your left hand to the big toe side of your foot. Allow your fingers on your top hand to point upwards. Be sure to do this pose on both sides.

To improve the pose:

- Look down at your foot or up at your hands — do whichever is more comfortable for you.

- The goal is to keep your shoulders parallel to one another.

- Use a block under your hand by your front foot to make your shoulders straighter and more aligned with each other.

- Press your feet strongly into the floor.

- Remember to twist through your spine, hands, shoulder and neck.

- Breathe strong!

Why should I do it?

This pose is challenging as it tests and strengthens your flexibility and strength. It also begins to test your balance because the twisting part of this pose requires you to pay attention to your feet and equilibrium: with all this on your mind, you'll have no room to feel mad about anything!

This pose also:

- Strengthens your ankles.

- Tones your legs.

- Helps keep the spine strong and released of tension.

- Energizes your entire body.

Half Lord of the Fishes Pose
(*Ardha Matsyendrasana*)

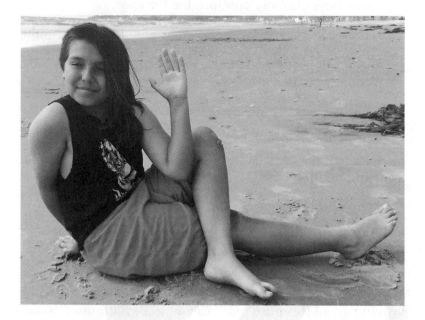

How do I do it?

Sit down comfortably. Keep your right leg straight out in front of your body and bend your left leg, crossing it over your right leg. Be sure your left foot is pressed in close to your right thigh. Reach your right arm up and twist your body over towards your bent left leg. If you can, rest your right elbow on the outside of the left leg. Bring your right hand directly behind you: pressing your wrist crease into the base of your spine, using your right arm as a "kickstand" keeping your entire spine straight. To come out of the pose, untwist slowly, coming back to center. Then switch your legs and twist to the other side.

To improve the pose:

- Make your spine straighter with each inhale.

- Twist deeper with each exhale.

- Relax your shoulders away from your ears.

- If you can't get your elbow to the opposite side of the knee, keep your arm straight (you'll get a great twist here too).

- Point or flex your extended foot.

- Use a block on the hand by your spine for support.

Why should I do it?

Twists detoxify the physical, emotional, and energetic bodies which will help you let go of anything causing negativity. What's extra great about this pose is that it provides this detoxification through sitting. This means you can do this pose at a chair in school or while you're watching TV or typing on a computer.

This pose also:

- Increases energy.

- Helps detoxify your body.

- Keeps your spine straight.

- Opens your chest and shoulders.

- Makes your torso more flexible.

- Makes your legs stronger.

Belly Twist
(*Jathara Parivartanasana*)

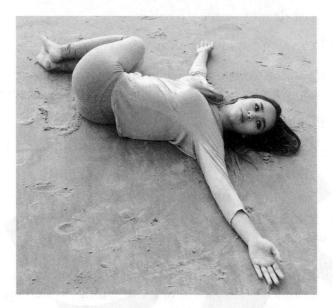

How do I do it?

Lay flat on your back. Bend your knees at a 90 degree angle. Spread your arms out wide to your sides. Drop your knees over to your right side; look over to your left side twisting your neck. When you are ready to unwind, twist back to center and move to the opposite side.

To improve the pose:

- Be sure to keep your shoulders down on the ground.

- Try to stack your knees on top of each other to get a deeper stretch.

- The closer you can bring your knees to your hip, the more intense the pose.

- To get a deeper stretch in your leg muscles, straighten your top leg out to the side.

- Breathe long inhales and exhales to help you twist better.

Why should I do it?

In this pose you are laying down, so you this provides a grounding and calming quality. With this, your lower body is twisting in one direction while your upper body is twisting in another direction. This symbolically encompasses the definition of being open-minded. Not only are you twisting to help let go of things energetically, but you are also moving your body in two different directions reminding you to see things from all sides. Having an open mind is a huge way to understand many things, and when you are understanding, you are less likely to experience anger and frustration. When you do this pose, let this lesson take over your body, mind, and soul.

This pose also:

- Opens your chest and heart (love cures anger!).

- Relaxes your neck.

- Makes your belly feel good (especially if you ate too much).

- Relaxes your body.

- Cools your body (making all that hot anger go away!).

Marchi's Pose
(*Marichyasana*)

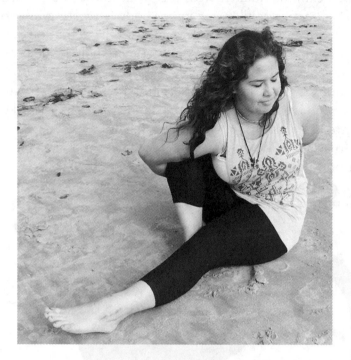

How do I do it?

Sit down with your legs straight out in front of you. Keep your right leg extended long and bend your left leg in. Keep the sole of your foot on the ground and try to bring your heel as close to your bottom as you can. Bend your left arm around you left knee. Fold forward. Reach your right arm behind you, trying to grab your left hand. If you can't reach your hand (not many people can!) hold a strap in each hand to stretch your arms properly. Be sure to do this pose on both sides of your body.

To improve the pose:

- Try different variations of this pose. There are four versions of this pose. Each version gets a little more difficult.

- Version A is what was discussed above.

- Version B consists of bringing the extended leg out into half lotus (resting your ankle upon your thigh).

- Version C consists of keeping the extended leg out but crossing it over the opposite thigh. From here, the arms are bound reaching for each other (use a strap if you can't reach your hands).

- Version D consists of combining B and D (so have that extended leg in half lotus and twist your arms binding your hands (again, a strap is helpful here!)

- No matter which version you do, always focus on your breath.

Why should I do it?

No matter what version of this pose, you are basically turning yourself into a twisted pretzel. I bet you've never seen a twisted man before have you? Seriously, "Marichi's Pose" is named after a great sage (a wise man) based on Hindu mythology. His name is translated as "the way of light." Because this posture is named after him, this pose teaches us to focus on attaining clarity instead of being blinded by anger and doing something regrettable.

This pose also:

- Increases your energy level.

- Helps detoxify your body.

- Gives your spine alignment (to improve your posture).

Revolved Chair Pose
(*Parivrtta Utkatnasana*)

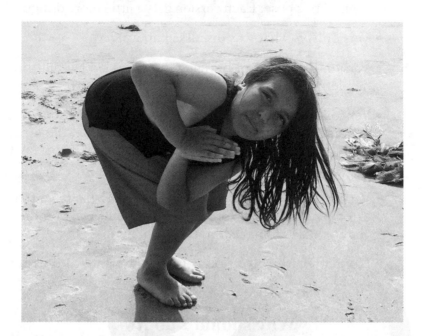

How do I do it?
Standing in Mountain Pose, bring your big toes to touch each other. Reach your arms up high above your head and begin to slightly squat, bending your knees as if you are sitting in a chair. Now bring your hand down to your heart in Anjali Mudra. Twist over to the right side, hooking your left elbow on the outside of the right knee. Continue bending into your knees. Be sure to twist on both sides of your body.

To improve the pose:

- Keep your hips facing forward, allowing the twist to come to the torso and belly (where all that anger energetically sits). To check to make sure you are doing this, make sure your knees are in line with one another. If one knee is peeking out in front of the other, bring the knee back into alignment. That will surely straighten out your hips.

- Lift your toes to make sure most of your weight is in your heels — this will help you "sit" back deeper into this pose.

- Really squeeze your knees together.

- Bring your shoulder back to open your chest more.

- Breathe in every time you twist deeper.

- You can separate your hands and stretch your arms open to get a deeper stretch.

Why should I do it?

You will absolutely feel this pose in your thighs! It's tough, but this pose reminds you to stand tall (keep your spine strong as you're twisting!) and breathe through any tension so you can twist deeper. This is pretty much the secret for dealing with anger: you have to be strong, endure discomfort and look at things from a different angle to release tensions. When you come out of the pose, you will feel energized and lighter. That is, too, exactly how you will feel when you let go of the anger in your life.

This pose also:

- Builds strength.
- Builds endurance.
- Makes the thighs stronger.
- Strengthens your balance.
- Makes your feet stronger.
- Detoxifies your body.

Breathing

Taking deep breaths will instantly make you feel less mad (and will keep you from saying and doing things that you will later regret). That's what anger does to us…it turns us in to someone who we really aren't.

The breath is super helpful here because when we are mad, the first thing that happens is we forget to breathe, then our heart rate starts to speed up, and our adrenaline starts to kick in… which can make us feel like a crazy monster! When we breathe, we slow down, our heart beats back at its normal rate, and we feel calm. This makes the angry monster we turned into start to go away.

However, there is a special breathing exercise designed just for controlling anger. This breathing exercise is thousands of years old! Let this remind you that everyone gets angry and people have been experiencing anger for thousands of years. It's all good. We just need to practice consciously to try our best to control it.

The Breath of Fire:

You are going to feel really funny doing this breath because it's not anything close to the normal breathing that we do (it's weird actually!) but you will definitely feel less angry after you do this exercise.

Here's how:

- Sit comfortably.

- Inhale (through your nose) sucking in your belly button.

- Exhale (through your nose) pushing out your belly (make yourself have a big gut!)

- Do this as fast as you can, creating a pumping action with your stomach.

Meditation

If I had to compare anger to one of the five elements, it would be fire. Anger is really fire within us that doesn't know how to be controlled. It even makes us hot (sometimes, if we are really mad, we will start to sweat!).

Think about a fire. If it is controlled, like in a fireplace or fire pit, or with a candle, it can bring us warmth, relax us, comfort us, and even inspire us. When it is not controlled, though, bad things can happen, and they can happen really quickly. An uncontrolled flame is destructive: it will burn and destroy all that it touches (and it does so without mercy or remorse, and it does not stop until a greater force comes in).

All of us have a flame within us. This is known as our "ego." Our ego is our level of worth and the value we put in ourselves. Basically, it's our self-confidence. When we feel confident, we are comforting and inspiring to others (and ourselves!) like a controlled candle flame. When we are agitated and our worth is threatened, this causes anger…which inflames into angry energy which can quickly cause destruction hurting ourselves and others around us. It is important to control our "flame."

With the permission and/or supervision of your parent or guardian, light a candle. Put the candle about 3-4 feet away from you at eye level. Gaze at this flame for as long as is comfortable for you. Don't strain your eyes, and be sure to stop when you feel you want to. As you look at this flame, take its controlled burning as inspiration. Meditate on being the controlled, burning light.

When you are done looking at the candle, blow it out, and blink your eyes closed for a few minutes (you will still see the flame!). Let this light inspire you to burn all that anger living deep inside of you.

When you open up your eyes, blink them open and shut for a little so your eyes can adjust to the natural lighting in the room.

Candle-gazing (known as Tatraka in Sanskirt) is a powerful yogi technique that is thousands of years old. It's very healthy for your eyes (especially for many teenagers like yourself who spend lots of time staring at electronics).

Be sure to ask for your parent's permission. They may ask why you are staring at a candle. Let them know it has a lot of health benefits. Aside from helping control anger, it:

- improves eyesight and vision.

- improves concentration, intelligence and memory.

- enhances self-confidence, patience and willpower.

- develops greater work efficiency and productivity.

- calms the mind and provides inner peace and silence.

- brings greater clarity with which we can make better decisions.

- helps to overcome mental, behavioral and emotional problems.

- provides stress relief and deep relaxation.

- deepens the sleep and helps sleep related disorders such as headache, insomnia, nightmares, etc.

- is much healthier than staring at a computer, TV, or cellphone screen.

Get your parents to meditate with you! If not or if they won't let you, don't get mad — it's no big deal. Just visualize a flame by closing your eyes and meditate by yourself.

Writing:

Meditative Writing AUMwork 1

Anger often occurs when stuff is held in. The more you push your feelings down inside, the more they will want to come up! Often times, when we hold in our feelings, this causes more frustration, until a point where we almost burst, just overflowing with emotion, and we end up getting really mad.

It can be really hard to have someone you can talk to about your anger. If you are brutally honest with your anger, others might not be able to understand you. Sometimes this can make you feel worse. This happened to me as a teen a lot. I felt like no one understood why I was mad, and that just made me more mad. After awhile, I got frustrated with people not understanding my anger, so I just didn't talk about it with anyone. All this anger built up in me, and then one day, I got so mad, I yelled, freaking out over something small to someone I really cared about!

Don't let things fester inside of you. You will burst with anger one day (like I did). Instead, keep a journal and write about all the anger you have. This will help you release any attachment you have to feelings or things that make you mad.

Paper is the best listener. Just write down all that makes you mad. There are no rules. Just write! You'll feel ten pounds lighter when you're done.

Meditative Writing AUMwork 2:

Anger also happens when we don't know how to explain or express our feelings. It is easier to get mad, yell, or be mean to others instead of facing what is really bothering us. Although this is easier, it is not good for us. Physically, our anger can turn into to tightness or pain. Being angry and not feeling good is no fun. Did you ever see a grumpy old man? You don't want to turn out like that.

When you're confused on your anger, try your best to answer the following question (I suggest answering through writing because writing allows our thoughts to be expressed more clearly than just speaking…especially when you are mad).

Think hard.
What is it that you are really getting mad at?

(Hint: Sometimes we act mad at something small, but really it's just getting blamed for something bigger, like when I was a teen I used to get so mad at my mom when she punished me, but really, I wasn't mad at her; I was mad at myself for doing something wrong that caused me to be punished in the first place.)

When you are done, crumble that paper up. Then, throw it out. Remember that you threw it out! You no longer need those thoughts: they are in the past, and they are gone. They are in the trash where they belong. Leave them there, and focus on having a peaceful, happy rest of your day.

Meditative Writing AUMwork 3
Anger can also happened instantly. We all have one negative emotion that we primarily express when we are a faced with something bad. For many teens, this is anger. Some people instantly get mad when something negative happens. When this happens people can yell or say things they don't mean. They can also get violent hurting themselves or others. Both of these negative reactions cause physical and emotional scars for all of the people involved.

Aside from using the breathing we talked about, writing can help. Change your habits. If you start this as a teen, dealing with anger will be so much easier as an adult. You will be a more mellow adult, for sure. When you feel that anger starting to erupt, breathe, then walk away. Instead of sitting with your thoughts or talking about them in a way that hurts others, use your writing. Grab a pen, and write about all that is making you mad: be brutally honest. Don't stop writing until you have said everything you need to. Then, to push the physical feelings away, rip up the paper! Tear it into a 100 little pieces. You will feel a lot better.

Chapter 5

Yoga for Love

Most of the songs on the radio are about some of form of love. Think about it. What is your favorite song? It's probably about love gone good or love gone bad or about something someone loves or doesn't love to do or be. Songs about cheating and anger are about love, too: they are just discussing the negative aspect of "love." I put "love" in quotes because pure love, true love, never is negative.

Most of the movies in theaters and shows on TV have love in them too: whether it be a show about relationships or families or a character or actor in a show doing something they love.

Love is everywhere! This is because love is everything. It is what keeps this world alive. Remember when we talked about the Sun Salutation and how it honors the heart, all that keeps us alive, our "sun?" Our heart represents love because life is love.

There are many forms of love. When most of us think about love, we think about soulmates or finding or being with our perfect person. We think about fairytales and being in a relationship or getting married! Although girls are more open with this thought, boys think about this too.

Love is limitless, so please remember this. Love is not just about soulmates, partners, and traditional relationships. If you don't have a boyfriend or girlfriend, it doesn't mean you don't have love. In fact, that couldn't be further from the truth.

Love is not about the physical either. Love exists without kissing or having sex. Being physical with someone will also not prove love. If you kiss or have sex with someone, and they (or you) are mean or unloving to that person that isn't a positive expression of love. Always remember that.

Love and matters of the heart get confusing. This is because love is so powerful. It can literally take our breath away! Most people have a conditional definition of love. They love their family because they have to. They look for love because they are told to. I'm here to tell you that love is so much more than that.

Love first starts with loving yourself. If you can't love and can't take of yourself, how will you know how to love and take care of other people? When people love others more than they love themselves, this causes a whole lot of imbalances and stress. Treat yourself with so much love, every day! When you're loving to yourself, the rest of the world will show you love too. I learned this first hand.

In my opinion, a perfect world is a world full of love. You are the future of this world, so live, learn, and teach other to being loving in every way, and realize, love is:

- **For everyone and everything**: you must love yourself and have love for all things. It is not segregated or judgmental. Love is pure.

- **Balanced**: Too much love will make you obsessive or jealous. Not enough love will make you scared or sad. Love in balance.

- **Fair**: Always be fair with love — love yourself as much as you love others. Love all things the same, in appropriate ways in which you decide.

- **Unconditional**: You can't love things based upon dictated expectations. There is no "I will love you if…" when it comes to love. Have some sort of love for all. Openly.

- **A practice**: With so many forms of love, and so many different perspectives on love, it can get confusing. Negativity can sometimes result of love too. Remember every day is a day to learn more and more about love, and if you make a mistake, it is ok. Send love to the mistake and keep learning!

These are big concepts for adults to understand and live, so if you are confused or overwhelmed with these definitions of love, don't worry, lots of people in the world are. That is why there is violence and killing and lots of other bad things. The world needs love. Teens are the future of the world, so be an example for love. Start by being nice and caring to yourself and everything and everyone around you (yes that includes your bratty brother or sister and even a spider).

Ultimately, no one can tell you what love is. You create your own definition of love based upon what your heart tells you, and yoga (stretching, breathing, meditating, writing, and hanging out with yourself) helps you come up with a clear definition.

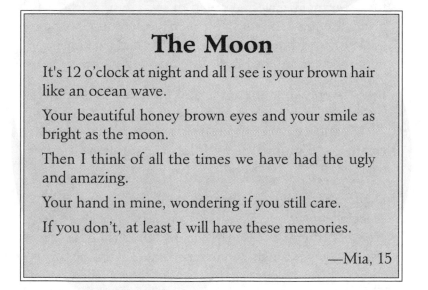

The Moon

It's 12 o'clock at night and all I see is your brown hair like an ocean wave.

Your beautiful honey brown eyes and your smile as bright as the moon.

Then I think of all the times we have had the ugly and amazing.

Your hand in mine, wondering if you still care.

If you don't, at least I will have these memories.

—Mia, 15

Stretches: Backbends

Backbends teach us to physically open our heart so we can let love in and give love to the world. The counter-balance or opposite of a backbend is a forward fold. If you ever feel too much love or overwhelmed by love, close your heart a little by folding forward. In the following the physical focus is on the heart, and when you physically focus on nurturing the heart, emotionally balance comes too.

Self-love is the most important love there is. You are on your own journey and your own path. No one else is going to live your story completely except for you. When we prioritize our heart chakra, we strengthen our 'self-love' muscle. You are with you for a long time, so it is really powerful to have unconditional love for yourself.

I have had glasses since kindergarten. Up until about 8th grade I was taller than 90% of the guys. I was skinny and lanky. At age 12, I had braces and a pallet expander that eventually gave me a gap in my teeth in which I could fit a straw through. But then having rubber bands hooked to my braces wasn't so bad as it closed my gap right up. I lacked much self-love and confidence.

I used to only know me as the dorky physical appearance that I felt like I was; not understanding at the time that my confidence comes from looking inward towards my creative and funny side and the free spirit that is my true self.

I believe everyone goes through an awkward stage in life especially during teen years. We can be kind if we are ever picked on or teased. That person teasing us may also be going through a confidence battle. The one thing we can control is our self-view, and what we believe our self-worth is. No one can give us that, not even all the compliments in the world. Because life happens, and it's up to ourselves to find contentment with where we are and who we are, here and now.

—Monica, 24

Cat-Cow Pose
(*Durga-Go*)

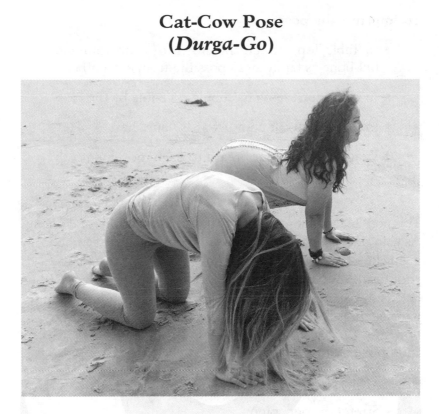

How do I do it?

Get stand on your hands and knees: this is called "Table Top Position." Be should your shoulders are directly under your wrists and your knees are directly under your hips. There are two parts of this pose. In the first part, Cat Pose, you suck your belly button in and press your hands firmly in the ground as if you are pressing the ground away from you. You make a C shape with your spine, tucking your chin and looking down, like a scared cat. In the second part, Cow Pose, drop your belly down, bring your shoulders back and your chest out while stretching your neck, looking up with your eyes (like a moo-ing cow). Take an inhale every time you do Cow Pose and exhale every time you do Cat Pose. Do as many rounds as you want.

To improve the pose:

- In Table Top, stretch the crown of your head and your tail-bone as far away as possible from each other.

- In Cow, don't let your shoulders come by the ears.

- In Cat, tuck your chin towards your chest.

- Really connect your breath to each movement.

Why should I do it?

This pose teaches how to love with your heart evenly and openly. As your open your chest in your Cow Pose, you are symbolically giving love to the world. As you draw your chest inward towards your head, you are energetically sending love to yourself. When love is in balanced: you equally have love and compassion for yourself and the world, your heart will be full and healthy.

This pose also:

- Tones your belly.

- Stretches your spine.

- Gives you energy.

- Warms up your muscles (good to do before lots of exercise!)

Cobra Pose
(*Bhujangasana*)

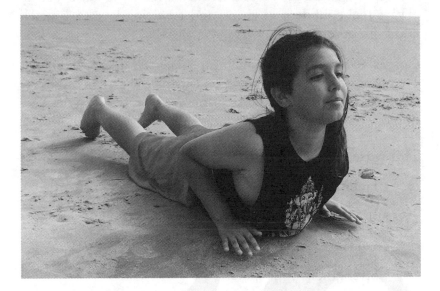

How do I do it?
Lay on your belly. Bring your arms by your side, pressing your hands into the ground even with your chest. Keep your toenails pressed into the floor and your legs pressed together. Lift your chest off the floor.

To improve the pose:

- Squeeze your elbows in to open your chest more.

- Never squeeze your gluts. Instead, suck in your belly.

- Allow your shoulders to come away from your ears.

- Don't worry about how high your chest is off the ground — the focus of this pose is a small, yet powerful backbend.

- Keep your leg muscles active.

- Close your eyes or look down at your nose.

- Breathe in every time you lift your chest higher off the ground.

- Put little or no weight in your hands.

Why should I do it?

This poses allows you to build your confidence (you need to use core strength to lift your chest), which will allow you to always feel confident in giving and receiving love to yourself and from others.

Cobras, too, are sacred animals especially in Hindu Mythology. They represent power, connection with all the chakras and they symbolism OM/AUM (the creation, preservation and destruction of everything).

This pose also:

- Helps make your back really flexible.

- Increases circulation in your lungs and belly.

- Opens your chest (making it easier to breathe!).

- Strengthens your spine.

- Stretches your shoulders.

- Energizes your legs.

Bow Pose
(*Dhanurasana*)

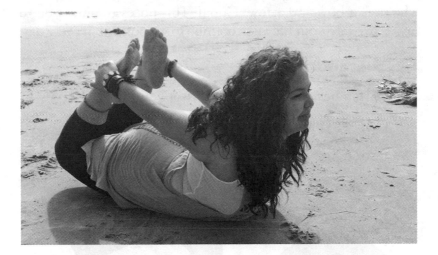

How do I do it?
Lay on your belly. Bend your legs towards your glutes. Reach around and grab the outside of your feet or ankles, slowly lifting your chest off the floor. You are making a "U" shape with your body.

To improve the pose:

- Really kick your legs/ankles into your hands. This will help your bend even more.

- Squeeze your shoulder blades close to each other to open your chest.

- Lift the top of your head higher and higher.

- Try to lift your thighs off the floor.

- Keep your knees inward. Inhale deeply as you open your chest more. Let your exhales keep you still and strong in the pose.

- Put a strap on the back of each foot and grab it with each hand allowing you to bend deeper.

Why should I do it?

Bow Pose represents a bow and arrow. Your torso is the bow and your arms represent the action of the bow string. Do you know who uses a bow and arrow? Cupid! This poses reminds you to invite love into your life and continue to welcome it in every day.

This pose also:

- Stretches the entire front part of your body.

- Opens your chest.

- Stretches your shoulders.

- Makes your neck strong.

- If you rock back and forth like a rocking horse you will massage your belly!

- Makes your lungs stronger (This is really good for people with asthma!).

Camel Pose
(*Ustrasana*)

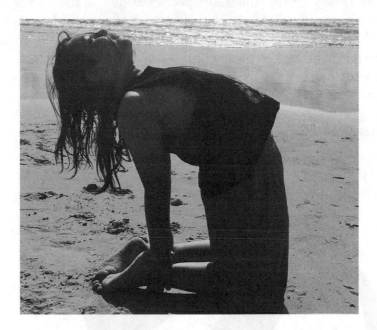

How do I do it?

Stand on your knees. Make two fists with your hands. Place them in between your thighs. This amount of space between your legs is known as "hip distance." With your knees hip distance apart, bring your hands to your backside as if they were going to go in imaginary back jean pockets! Squeeze your elbows towards one another, and with strength begin to stretch your neck back. As you backbend, keep your hips and knees even with one another.

To improve the pose:

- To make this pose more difficult, begin to bring your hands to your ankles or heals. If you can't reach them, come high on your toes. Be sure to keep your hips and knees in a straight line.

- Relax your neck.

- Look up (stretching your eyes).

- Focus on your breath here as with your throat open and your face back, breathing will be more difficult.

Why should I do it?

If you are scared of love or opening your heart, this pose is for you! This is a very vulnerable pose that allows you to release any blockages you may have in your heart (from past heartache) and be open for love again. This is a perfect pose to do when you feel heartbroken or unworthy to give love. It will teach you how to open your heart and let love in. If you already open with love, this will keep inviting love in your life!

This pose also:

- Strengthens your thighs.

- Invigorates your chest.

- Stretches your ankles.

- Increases circulation in your throat.

- Strengthens your back.

Royal Pigeon Pose
(*Rajakapotasana*)

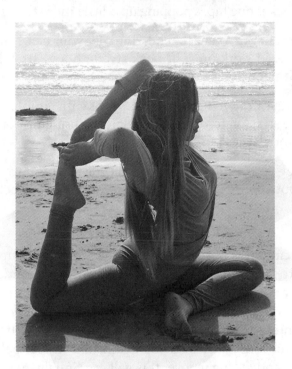

How do I do it?

From Table Top Pose, bring your right knee up to your chest. Place your right foot on the floor to the outside of your left leg. Bring your right knee to the outside of your right hand. Lower the outside right leg to the floor. Stretch your left leg back behind you. Lower your hips to the ground. Then, bend your left knee and reach back for the foot. The "complete pose" is when you have your foot touching the back of your head (don't force this! This takes lots of time and practice. I still can't do this.) Take your time releasing your arms and legs to come out of this pose. Do the same thing with your other leg.

To improve the pose:

- Keep your hips completely even in this pose. Sit on a block if one hip is popping up a little more than the other.

- Whenever you backbend, don't let your head fall back — instead work on your neck strength and stretch it back with control.

- Use a strap to help grab your foot with your hand. Hook the strap on to your foot and grab it bringing both of your hands over your head.

- Let your mind and body relax. Breathe into the tight spots. Remember, where ever you are is perfect

Why should I do it?

Energetically, this pose does two things: opens the hips (allowing you to let go of past hurt as the hips are energetic storage places for past pain) and opens the heart allowing in new love. If you can't get over something or someone, or feel stuck in love, living in memories of the past, do this pose. It will help release and open your heart up again. If you feel balanced in letting go and letting in love, this will continually help you stay healthy and strong.

This pose also:

- Brings flexibility in your hips: which is super helpful when you are stuck sitting for long periods of time.

- Stretches the muscles in your belly.

- Makes your hips stable.

- Open yours chest.

- Strengthens your spine.

Fish Pose
(*Matsyasana*)

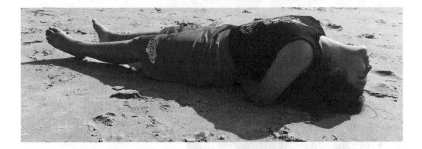

How do I do it?

Lay on your back. Sit on the top of your hands. Squeeze your elbows inward as you come to the top of your head. Your chest, ribs, and throat should be lifted.

To improve the pose:

- Rest a block in between your shoulder blades to help you get on your head.

- Place a blanket under your head for comfort.

- Flex your feet.

- Breathe deep from your lifted chest.

- Play with different versions in this pose:

- Cross your legs into Lotus Pose.

- Bring your hands to Anjali Mudra in front of your heart.

- Lift your arms and legs straight out in front of you.

Why should I do it?

Because you are resting on your head in this pose, not only are you opening your heart in this pose, you are also activating your belief center. Because of this, this pose will help you believe in love again (just in case you lost it) or keep you connecting with your faith in terms of love and compassion.

This pose also:

- Increases circulation in your throat (you'll speak more clearly! Good to do before public speaking).

- Stretches the ribcage.

- Improves digestion.

- Stretches your belly.

- Strengthens your back.

- Helps with breathing issues.

Bridge Pose
(*Setu Bandhasana*)

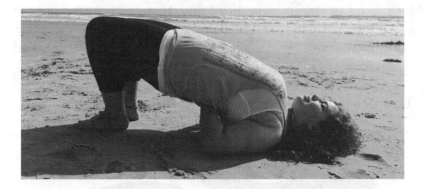

How do I do it?

Lay on your back bending your knees and bringing them as close to your hips as you can. The goal is to have your fingertips be able to graze the back of your heels. Bend your elbows into the ground with your hands facing up (your arms should feel like a robot). On your next inhale, lift your hips up as high as you can. You can keep your arms where they are or interlace your hands behind your back, coming up on your shoulders. You can also bring your hands to the small of your back helping to support you in this pose.

When you want to come down, do so with an exhale. Slowly come down vertebrae by vertebrae you glutes the last thing to touch the floor. Keep your spine neutral for a few breaths.

To improve the pose:

- Press your feet really firm into the ground.

- With each inhale, bring your hips up higher.

- Place a block under your tail-bone and let your body's weight be held by the block for a more restorative version.

- Bring your hips only as high as feels good.

Why should I do it?

This pose is an amazing way to open your heart without going into a full backbend (Wheel Pose), which can be scary and takes a lot of strength and flexibility. It is great practice to get you physically ready for Wheel Pose, and emotionally and energetically ready to continually open your heart and let love and compassion fulfill every part of you.

This pose also:

- Helps get rid of feelings of sadness or depression.

- Relieves any back tightness.

- Gets rid of menstrual cramps.

- Stretches your belly.

- Strengthens your spine.

- Opens your chest.

- Increases circulation in your Thyroid Gland (which works with your metabolism).

Wheel Pose
(*Urdhva Dhanurasana*)

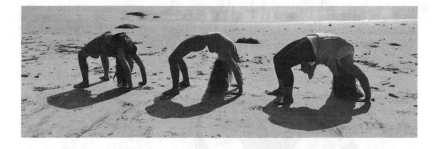

How do I do it?

Laying on your back, bend your knees and bring your heels as close as you can to your hips. Place your hands on the floor, under your shoulders, your fingers pointing toward your feet. Picture your spine really long and straight. Press your feet and hands firmly against the floor and on an inhale, lift your body up to the crown of your head. Stay here for your exhale. On your next inhale, left open your chest, and then on your exhale straighten your arms and legs lifting your head off the ground. You are making a rainbow shape with your entire body. Stay here as long as feels comfortable letting your breath support you.

To come out of the pose, move slowly. Slowly rest down on the top of the head on an exhale, and then bring each vertebrae down to the floor. Keep your spine neutral for a few breaths.

To improve the pose:

- Focus on maintaining balance between the weight in your hands and your feet.

- Let the head hang with strength and control.

- Breathe!

Why should I do it?

This pose opens up everything. It is also known as "Chakra Pose" because all of the energy circles in your body are being invigorated in this intense backbend. This means you'll be more grounded, fearless, confident, loving, truthful, intuitive, and connected to your beliefs! This is one of the most energetically powerful poses in yoga.

This pose also:

- Increases your flexibility.

- Strengthens pretty much everything: your shoulders, arms, wrists, legs, spine.

- Increases your energy.

- Shows you the world from a new view.

- Opens your chest (helping improve breathing issues).

- Makes you feel light and free.

Breathing

If love could be associated with one of the five elements, it would be air. You have heard of "falling in love." This is because we fall without anything but air (hope) holding us!

Air brings life. We breathe air every second, and this is what keeps us alive. Love works the same way. All forms of love keep us alive.

Air also brings lightness and freedom. In the same, when we experience love for ourselves, others, and all things, we are free from negative thoughts and emotions like hate, fear, anger, and sadness. We feel light!

Bring your hand on your heart. Breathe in as much air as possible. Feel your heart fill up with air. Remember that air is love. Exhale this air (this love) giving it back to the world. Keep doing this, sending lots of love and air to your body. Stop when you feel filled with love!

Meditation

A really powerful way to learn love is to meditate on your beating heart. Your heart literally loves you: unconditionally. It beats for you regardless of the day and time. If you eat a ton of junk food, it still loves you. It gives to you every second you are alive. This is love.

Meditate on your heart

Here's how:

- Sit comfortably.

- Close your eyes.

- Put your hands over your heart, feel it beating.

- Let each beat teach you love.

- Remember love is constant and giving.

- Meditate on your heart space for as long as you feel comfortable, trying to meditate for at least 10 minutes a day.

Writing

Meditative Writing AUMwork 1

Write love letters. Not just to a person you love, but to everyone and everything! Try writing a love letter to a tree—tell it you love it for all the fresh oxygen it brings you. It sounds kind of weird to write love letters to anything and everything like trees (society tells us romance and love is only for one person!) but love and compassion is universal, and everyone and everything deserves love. You will feel more love by giving love to all things too. This exercise will also help you understand that love is not a conditional or segregated thing. It is also not something to be afraid of.

Meditative Writing AUMwork 2

Expressing love to your friends, family, and boy/girl friend is pretty easy. The true test is learning how to be loving to bad things, events or people. To do this, you have to have compassion. Compassion is having a deep sympathy for someone or something that is expressing or experiencing negativity. It is consciously understanding that everything deserves love and those things and events that aren't loving, aren't because love was lacking from somewhere in his/her/its life.

The world needs compassionate people. Write on what compassion means to you. How can you show it? Why should you show it? Is it hard for you? Why? Think about how you can apply this to your life.

The first reaction to negative situations or people is the opposite of love. No one loves cancer or car accidents. Not many people love Hitler or murderers. Not many people love feeling lonely or different. I don't love these things, but I do have lots of compassion for them in my heart.

When I was in middle school, my Pop-pop (grandfather) died of cancer. I hated cancer, and I hated that he died and left making everyone super sad.

When I was in high school, my parents got divorced, and my dad started dating a new woman. Although he is married to her now, I hated her. I hated everything about my family being torn apart and different than it was my whole life. I hated hearing my parents talk badly about each other, and I hated coming home.

Yoga has taught me that hate just makes me feel bad. It makes my body not feel so good, and it makes me make bad decisions. When something negative is happening, we have the choice to make it better or worse. Always choosing love will make it better.

As an adult, I now know compassion. I still don't love cancer or divorce, but I do consciously accept it, feel for it, and send it love. Compassion allows me to be understanding, and through understanding something, positive thinking happens.

I send compassion to my Pop-pop's death: he lived for 77 years, and he found true love and had a bunch of kids, one of which grew up and had me. He had a happy life and was barely sick throughout it.

I have compassion for the cancer that killed him: it didn't torture him for decades: he could have suffered for a long, long time.

I also have compassion for the sadness my family and I all felt (and still feel) now that he is gone. Feeling sad over the loss of a person means you miss this person—and you can only miss something you love! How lucky am I and my family to have loved my Pop-pop and all the greatness he was! He's still alive within me today (you're reading about him right now!).

I send compassion to my parent's divorce. It taught me to accept change and see love in a different way. It has invited new people in my family. When I saw divorce through hate, I felt loss. Now that I see divorce through compassion, I see how much my family and I have gained.

It would have been powerful if I really understood compassion when I was a teen: I'd be an even better adult today and the days of my past would have been a lot happier.

How did I learn this? I just shifted my definition of love. Write about this. How can you shift your definition? How can you love that bad stuff in your life and this world?

Meditative Writing AUMwork 3
The last part of love to understand is fear. Most of us don't love as good as we can because we are afraid. We are afraid of rejection or being left. We are afraid of not being good enough or not being happy.

Here's a couple things to reflect upon in your writing:

Self Love:
Being in a relationship or being in love will not make you happy. It hopefully will make you happier, but it will not "cure" you or instantly make you a happy person. You become a blissful person by loving yourself. Do you love yourself? If you do, what does this mean? How can you continue to love yourself more and more everyday? How can you teach others to love themselves too? If you don't, why don't you? What can you do to love yourself? How can you shift the feelings of unlove for yourself and realize you are awesome and deserve so much self love (because you do—everyone does)?

Jealously and Obsession:
Do you get mad or jealous when you aren't getting enough attention from the people you love? What do you do? Yell at them? Pick fights? How do these things not help your heart?

Do you constantly think about a person over and over? Is that all you can think about? Why? How could this be a problem? How could you fix it?

Conditional Love:

Do you love conditionally? Do you only love a person if they act a certain way or wear certain clothes or look a certain way? This isn't pure love: it is superficial. You are hiding behind things or expectations instead of being open and loving. Why are you doing this? Why is this wrong? How can you change this?

Fear:

Most people—adults especially—don't have enough love in their life because they are scared of it. They are scared to ask for it because they feel they will be rejected or left. They are scared to invite it in their life because they are afraid of change. A lot of the time, these fears start as a teenager, when people have their first crush, boy/girlfriend, and kiss. Can you relate to this? If you do, try not to be scared: if you get rejected, you tried! If your life changes, it will be for the better. Reflect on all of this, and then answer the following questions:

How can you not be afraid of love? How can you inspire the world to be less fearful and more loving?

Chapter 6

Yoga for Patience

Being patient can be one of the hardest things in the world. I remember my parents always telling me to "be patient" and I wanted to scream: I hate waiting! I wanted what I wanted immediately.

If you can relate to this, then you know my pain (and I know yours!). I feel like all I remember doing as a teen was waiting! I'd wait for the time to run out in the classes that bored me; I couldn't wait for the weekends and to hang out with my friends. When I had my first love, Mikey Hickman, the minutes would literally feel like hours until I would see him again. I hated waiting for my parents to pick me up or drop me off; I couldn't wait until I could drive myself around. I couldn't wait for summertime, and I wanted nothing else but to be a grown up and not have to follow curfew. The worst waiting game of all was waiting for my college acceptance letters; that was just pure torture.

Waiting and waiting is a bad habit to get into. Why? It puts our brain in the state of never being satisfied. This causes us stress: it makes us super antsy and always wanting and wondering as opposed to being and living.

Many of you, though, may have the opposite of this problem. We live in a society that is so fast! If you want pretty much anything, you can find it or get it with just a click of a button. This creates a very urgent society that doesn't have to wait, and if you don't really have to wait, then you don't really learn how to appropriately handle waiting when you're forced to do it. Waiting and being patient could be a completely new concept for you.

If you're not a very patient person or you never learned to be patient, don't worry. You can learn anything and change any negative emotional trait you possess, and noticing you are this way is the first step. Breathing, meditating, and hanging out in calming, slow seated poses really helps slow down the active mind that wants, wants, wants, and transitions it to a mind happy exactly where it is.

If you are a patient person, teach other teens how to be this way! A patient adult is pretty much one of the best characteristics you can have because it leads to so many other positive emotional traits like being understanding, happy, peaceful, present, grounded, and appreciative.

Stretches: Seated and Restorative Poses

There are many types of yoga: some yoga is super fast and sweaty and other types are slow and calming. Moving slow and doing poses that are slow is a really good way to develop a patient mind.

All of the following poses will help you slow down. Try holding these poses for at least one minute (but try making a goal to eventually hold each pose for ten minutes!). This is how I learned patience (and remind myself of it every day). Just hang out there in the pose, patiently, and let your body release tension and receive all of the benefits the pose has to offer.

Lotus Pose
(*Padmasana*)

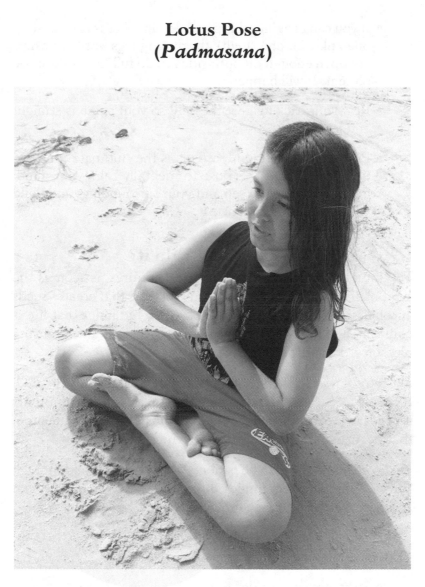

How do I do it?

Sit with your legs crossed. Cross each ankle over the opposite thigh. You can bring your hands to a mudra!

To improve the pose:

- Try sitting on a block: it will lift your hips up and may make this pose more accessible.

- If you can't get into this pose, do Half-Lotus (only resting one ankle on one thigh) alternating legs until your hips are open enough on both sides to do full Lotus Pose. Be patient. It will happen!

- Rest your back against the wall so your spine is straight and long.

- Practice meditating here. This is the "ultimate" meditation pose, so use this pose to mentally calm your mind, be patient with yourself and your surroundings and build your meditation practice.

Why should I do it?

The lotus, a beautiful flower, in many cultures, is seen as the symbol of karma. It is one of the only flowers that creates seeds and blossoms at the same time. This is a reminder that life is constant, and for every cause (the seed), there is an effect (the blossom). This is the definition of karma.

The lotus flower is also one of the only flowers that grows in mud. It is only from these murky waters that it can gain the nutrients it needs to create both seeds and blossoms. It is a reminder, too, that beauty sometimes must endure murk.

This pose reminds you to be patient: live with karma and through karma. When life gets muddy, be patient: a flower will bloom and new seeds are already growing.

This pose also:

- Stretches your ankles.

- Helps with tightness in your hips and knees.

- Helps you feel balanced.

- Increase circulation.

- Gives you energy

Child's Pose
(*Balasana*)

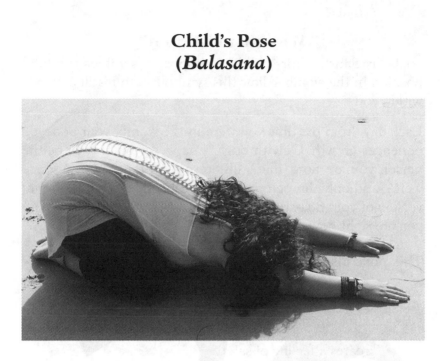

How do I do it?

From a kneeling position, sit down on your heels. Then, on an exhale, fold forward, resting your forehead on the ground, walking your hands as far out in front of you as you can.

To improve the pose:

- Focus on stretching through this movement by sitting back on your heels while reaching out with your arms.

- Roll your forehead back and forth, massaging it (and your third eye!)—it'll make you better with your intuition).

- Breathe!

Try a different version to stretch things differently:

- Spread your knees wide and have your big toes touch

- Rest your hands down by your side

- Bring your hands in Anjali Mudra and bend your elbows, resting your hands on the back of your neck.

Why should I do it?

"Bala" is Sanskrit for "child." This pose resembles the fetal position in the womb. Allow this symbolism to instill patience within you.

Each day, from the time you were in the womb, your body experiences growth. Only through time were you able to be the person you are now (much different than the fetus you once were), and only through time will you be able to be the future version of you. Be patient with growth and enjoy exactly where you are right now.

This pose also:

- Restores energy.

- Calms the mind (try this before a big test or game!).

- Creates a feeling of safety.

- Relaxes your neck and shoulders.

- Helps with digestion (good for when you eat junk food!).

Seated Forward Bend
(*Paschimottanasana*)

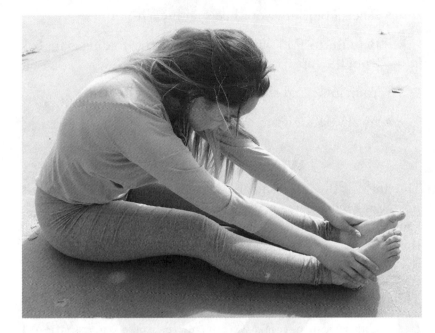

How do I do it?

From a seated position, straighten your legs out in front of you. Be sure to keep your spine really straight, then on your exhale fold forward. As you bend, keep your back straight. Reach for your feet, allowing your hands to fall where ever they go.

To improve the pose:

If your legs are tight:

- bend your knees

- rest your head on a block

- allow your hands to fall on your knees

- use a strap around your feet

- sit on a block or blanket

If your legs are very open:

- Interlace your hands around your heels

- Place a block by your heels and reach

- Be sure to fold with a flat back. The folding happens from the hips.

- Your spine and shoulders shouldn't be hunched.

- As always, don't forget to breathe.

Why should I do it?

The muscles in your body are very versatile. You can hold this pose for a while, and it will be safe as long as you take your time. Use props or slowly adjust your body as you hang out in this pose. Take your time and notice the longer you are here, the deeper you will be able to fold.

This pose also:

- Calms your nervous system (nerves make you impatient).

- Helps you digest what you have eaten throughout the day.

- Helps get rid of tiredness.

- Can help make headaches go away.

Wide-Angle Seated Forward Fold
(*Upavishtha Konasana*)

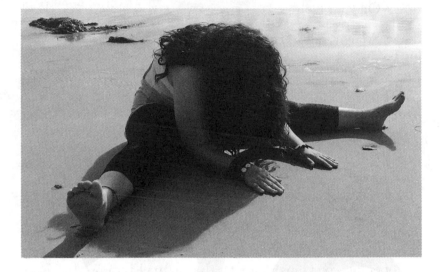

How do I do it?
This pose is a straddle pose. From a seated position, stretch out your legs as wide as you comfortably can. Then, fold towards the floor. When you want to come out of this pose, slowly raise up with your heart and bend both of your legs inward.

To improve the pose:

- Fold from your hips.

- Keep your toes pointed up so your legs are active.

- On your exhales, challenge yourself to fold deeper.

Rest your hands:

- By your ankles

- On your feet/toes

- Straight out in front of you

- On blocks

- In a mudra

- Anywhere else that feels comfortable

Why should I do it?

You probably do a whole bunch of sitting in school (and you probably want to get up A LOT. How could you not be impatient if you're stuck at a desk all day?). This pose will help make sitting easier for you! Although you are seated in this pose, you are opening your hips in a way that actually counterbalances traditional sitting. This is so important because if we don't give our body the opposite of what it always does, tension builds up. Lots of tension makes it hard to sit, and having a hard time sitting totally makes a person impatient.

This pose also:

- Opens your hips.

- Stretches all the muscles in your legs.

- Helps with digestion.

- Stretches your arms.

- Makes your inner thighs feel good.

Bound Angle Pose
(*Baddha Konasana*)

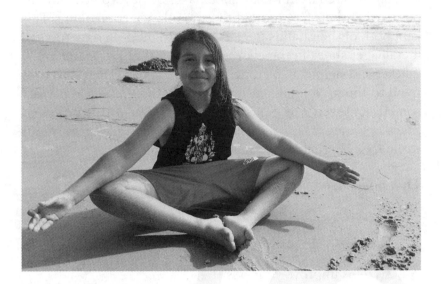

How do I do it?

From a comfortable seat, bring both of the soles of you feet together. Sit up straight with your spine long. Be patient and enjoy this pose. When you come out of it, use your hands to help close your knees inward.

To improve the pose:

- To help you sit straight, sit against a wall.

- Place blocks under each knee if you feel uncomfortable.

- The closer you bring your ankles to your body, the more stretch you will bring to your hips (this is good if you sit for long periods of time).

- The further you bring your ankles away from your body, the more stretch you will get on your ankles (this is good if you walk or run a lot!).

Why should I do it?

Each of the poses were taken from India's history. This pose was actually inspired from Indian shoemakers. They would sit in this pose, using their feet to hold the shoe they were making. This kept both of their hands free. Take this to modern day. You can literally get shoes in the click of a button that are made much quicker and simpler in factories! Appreciate this. Then shift your mind to things you create: it takes time to carefully construct something (even if it is just a thought!). Sit in this pose and practice patience. It will help you honor the quickness of our world today and also the creator within you.

This pose also:

- Stretches the thighs.

- Increase circulation (which gives you energy).

- Helps improve your posture.

- Makes your hips and thighs less tight.

Half Splits
(*Hanumanasana*)

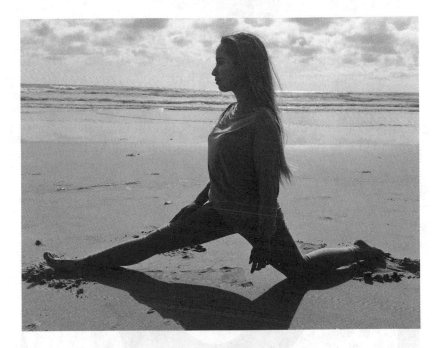

How do I do it?

Begin in a kneeling lunge: starting in table top position, bring your right leg forward. Place your hands on the sides of your feet. Begin to straighten your right leg, pressing your heel into the ground. Your toes should be pointing back to your face. Fold forward from your hips.

To improve the pose:

- Bring blocks under both of your hands to help you fold with a flat back.

- With patience, work on coming into a full split where both of your legs are straightened—one foot forward pointing, another foot backwards pointing.

- Sit on a block, helping you straighten both of your legs out to a full split.

- No matter where you are, take full breaths to help loosen any muscles in the legs. This will help you get deeper in the pose.

Why should I do it?

This pose is inspired by the Hindu Mythology of Hanuman, the magical flying monkey. Legend has it he took a great leap (making the split posture!) to help rescue the wife of a famous lord.

This pose is very difficult (as is helping others.) Let this pose remind you to be patient, and that great leaps take time.

This pose also:

- Release tightness in your legs.

- Helps your hips feel good.

- Makes your spine strong.

- Works out your stomach muscles.

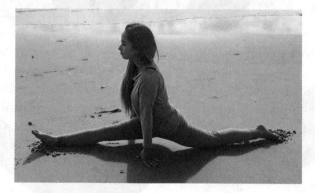

Corpse Pose
(*Savasana*)

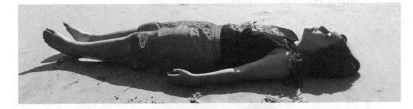

How do I do it?

Lay flat on your back. Allow your legs and feet to rest wherever and however they want. Lay still, completely relaxed yet fully aware.

To improve the pose:

- Allow your breath to be natural.

- Don't fall asleep: the point of this pose is to be awake but 100% relaxed.

- Rest a bolster or rolled up blanket under your knees (this is helpful if your back is achy).

- Place a blanket over your body to stay warm (your body temperature drops when you are still).

- Place a blanket under your head to be comfortable.

- Close your eyes or use an eye pillow to block out distracting lights.

Why should I do it?

It is a true test to be completely relaxed but not fall asleep! Most people have lots of thoughts going through their head: their mind is like a ball bouncing from one thought to the next. Coming to a place where your mind is completely still and present, and your body is completely relaxed may take time. Be patient. The stillness and awareness will come!

This pose also:

- Completely relaxes your physical and mental body.
- Calms your emotions.
- Helps you feel present.
- Relieves tensions.

Breathing

Slowing down and breathing will immediately help you become more patient, so try your hardest to focus on your breathing when you get impatient. There is also a very old, sacred breathing technique known as Nadi Shodhana, which translates to: Alternate Nostril Breathing. Doing this breathing exercise may seem a little odd (it is not a normal, everyday type of breathing), but after a few rounds, you will notice that antsy-ness caused by impatience will start to fade away as this breathing exercise really focuses on centering the mind's activity.

Here's how:

- Sit comfortably.

- Place your left hand on your left knee. You can just let your hand rest comfortably or use the ancient mudra (hand symbol) taught with this pose, Cin Mudra, where you place your index finger and thumb to gently touch at the tips.

It looks like this:

Then...

- Place the tip of your index finger and middle finger of your right hand in between the eyebrows. Place your little finger on your left nostril and your thumb on your right nostril.

- Press the thumb down on the right nostril and breathe out of your left nostril.

- Breathe in through your left nostril.

- Press the left nostril closed with your little finger.

- Remove the right thumb from the right nostril and breathe out from the right.

- Breathe in from the right, and then exhale from the left.

- This is one complete round of Alternate Nostril Breathing. Complete as many rounds as you need to feel patient and calm!

Meditating

A really powerful way to learn patience is by experimenting with your breath. Holding your breath for as many counts as you inhale and exhale will allow your lung capacity to build (which will allow you to subconsciously and naturally take deeper and fuller breaths which will help you to be physically and mentally healthier). Holding your breath, too, will teach you patience.

Here's how:

Note: It is not safe or healthy to hold your breath to a point where you feel weird, dizzy or even start to see spots or black. Do not ever do this.

You are going to count your breaths (or have someone count your breathing) so focus is practiced in this breathing exercise as well.

Start by counting to three.

- Take an inhale for 3 counts.

- Hold your breath for 3 counts.

- Exhale for 3 counts.

- Keep inhaling, holding, and exhaling in this way. If three seems too easy, increase your count. Safely challenge yourself.

Writing

Meditative Writing AUMwork 1:
Do you consider yourself a patient person? If you said yes, how can you help others be patient? If you said no, what are some things you can do to be more patient?

Meditative Writing AUMwork 2:
Reflect on this simple question: Why is it important to be patient?

Meditative Writing AUMwork 3:
A peaceful life is one where the person is not waiting, but being in the present moment! Think about the things that make you impatient. How can you change your mind from a place of waiting to a place of being?

Chapter 7

Yoga for Fear

A lot of people, generally, hide their fear because they see it as a sign of weakness. Society gives us this impression. Movies and sport games, for example, glorify being tough and wrongly call this "strength." As a result, we believe we need to be seen as tough so we shouldn't experience fear because if we do, someone might think of us as fragile or a baby. This is the absolute opposite of the truth: a person who admits their fears and then faces them is a person who has true strength. Unfortunately, a lot of the times, the world doesn't see it this way.

As a teen, I was scared of so many things, but because I didn't want to look like a "baby," I hid my fear. I replaced it with by not dealing with this emotion and trying to act cool or tough. To act this way, I just shoved all that fear far away so I (and no one else) could see it.

When Mikey broke up with me (one of the 1,4567 times!) I acted like I didn't care (really I was scared to death I would never be loved again!)

When I got a bad grade on a test, I hid it (because I was too scared to show my parents because I didn't want them to think I wasn't smart).

When my friends were all shoplifting at the mall, I was too scared to admit I didn't want to do it, so I stole some clothes and got arrested. Scared to death in a cop car and so ashamed of what I did, I still acted like it didn't bother me.

And then, when I turned 19 and went to college, and my friends asked me to go to a frat party in a bad neighborhood, I fearlessly said yes, only to get mugged at gun point! This left me scared to death, but I never really talked about this fear with anyone or did anything healthy to deal with it. Instead, I locked myself in my dorm room and didn't go out in the city for six months! Instead of telling my friends why, I made up excuses.

This denial of fear followed me well into my twenties. I kept this habit with me. I was scared to express my feelings to others and talk about important things that were going on in my life. I was scared to say "no" when I didn't want to do something, and I was scared to just be me (we will talk about self-confidence in the next chapter because fear and confidence go hand in hand).

This pushing away of fear got me to be a very, very anxious twenty-three year old who had panic attacks regularly. The most ironic thing of all was that I was too scared to tell anyone that this was happening to me (I didn't want anyone to think I was weak or feel bad for me!) so I ignored them for a couple more years until I got sick with severe anxiety disorder and couldn't ignore it anymore. This anxiety disorder is what led me to yoga (and I am so grateful for that) but I know, if I would have talked about my fears openly as a teenager, I wouldn't have had to deal with it as an adult.

Anything and everything can be scary to a person: we create our own illusions and fears in our heads. No one can tell you your fear is not valid. In the same, you can't tell anyone that you have never experienced fear.

I have worked with a lot of teens over the years helping them cope with anxiety. I know teens have experienced fears in so many different areas. Most common has been teens dealing with fears associated with having sex, their future, learning to drive, school and peer pressure. I have helped teens deal with big fears from death or fear caused after the loss of a loved one, to something not as big (but equally as important as any and all fears matter) like not being asked to the prom.

From my personal experience being a teen and working with teens, I know there's a lot of stuff that goes on in middle and high school that is straight up scary. I once taught yoga to a girl's volleyball team to help relax them before their biggest game of the year. One of the girls told me she always gets so nervous before the games that she actually throws up. This story is normal, actually, as most people don't know how to deal with their fears in a healthy way, so they feel it physically. Positively, fear doesn't have to win because yoga gives insight on how to beat it.

Stretches: Balancing Poses

To get over fears, you have to face your fears, but you have to do this in a smart and logical way. For example, if a person is deathly afraid of flying in an airplane, jumping out of an airplane may not be the best solution. Taking baby steps is a better way to deal with anxiety.

With this, fear also causes an imbalance in your mind. You are too much in the "fight or flight" mode as opposed to a state of mental calm and relaxation. This happens because the brain is thinking way too much. There is no balance.

A way to develop balance in the mind is to create balance in the body. Practicing balancing poses will literally lessen the weight of the thoughts in your head: it is impossible to hold a balancing pose if you are worrying. These poses force you to stay in the present moment, and when you are focused on what you are doing, you will be fearless. Anxiety only happens when we are thinking about the past or future.

Last, be sure to start slow: take baby steps! Try the easier poses like Tree Pose and Side Plank before getting into more difficult poses like Crow or Crane.

Balancing Tips:
There are six secrets to balancing properly without falling over.

Here they are:

1. Have a strong foundation: make sure your feet (or hands, depending on what pose you are doing) are planted firmly on the floor.

2. Have a strong core (you core connects with your confidence—think about your Third Chakra), so suck in your belly and believe in yourself.

3. Keep your chest open and your spine straight. Use this symbolism as inspiration: an open heart will allow you to experience things you never thought you could.

4. Look at something that is not moving. When your gaze (or "Dristi" as written in Sanskrit) is focused, you are less likely to fall over.

5. Empty your mind. Thoughts bring heaviness, and to balance, you need to be mentally as light as a feather!

6. Don't be afraid to use support! Use a wall or another person to help you with your balance. Then experiment with practicing the poses without the support of others. You can do it!

Tree Post
(*Vrkshasana*)

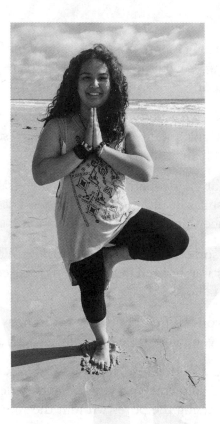

How do I do it?
From Mountain Pose, ground into your right foot and bring
your hands to center pressing them into one another. Begin to
lift your left foot up, then bring your knee outwards and finally
press your sole of your foot on the inner part of right leg (either
above the ankle or knee—never rest your foot on joints). If you
feel stable here, begin to raise your arms over your head. Try
to hold this pose for a few breaths. When you feel you want to
come out of it, bring your hands down first, followed by your
leg. Be sure to do the opposite side.

To improve the pose:

- Create positive friction between your foot and leg: press the sole of the foot into the side of the leg; press the side of the leg into the sole of the foot.

- Remember the 6 balancing tips!

- Breathe, keeping your chest open and full.

- Close your eyes if you want more of a challenge.

- If you are having trouble with balance:

- Adjust where you place your foot. Your foot can rest right on top of your ankle.

- Use a friend to help keep you balanced.

- Hold on to the wall to keep you balanced.

- Practice different expressions with your arms:

- Bring your hands to any mudra you know.

- Stretch your arms over to each side for a side body stretch.

- Come up with your own arm expression!

Why should I do it?

Fear stems from a place of disconnect. Many times when people are dealing with anxiety, it is because they are in their heads as opposed to being focused on the present moment. This ungroundedness feeds anxiety. Tree Pose reminds us to be present and grounded, and from this, fear will disappear.

Use the symbolism of a tree to deal with anxiety. Trees don't have any control of their destiny: animals inhabit it, weather messes with it, and humans cut trees down. The total trust and wisdom a tree represents is the key to removing fear from your life.

When standing in Tree Pose, allow your foot to represent the roots: strong and stable. Allow your arms to represent the branches continually growing. If you sway, it's ok: trees sway, too. Release fear as you surrender and use the stability of this pose to calm the instability of fearful thoughts.

This pose also:

- Makes your legs strong.

- Builds concentration.

- Improves focus.

- Makes your ankles more stable.

- Opens your hips.

- Increases your overall body strength.

Eagle Pose
(*Garudasana*)

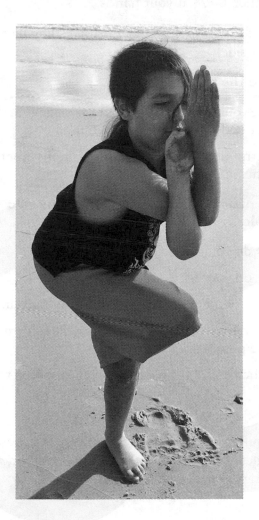

How do I do it?

Come into Chair Pose: bring your hands down to your heart in Anjali Mudra. Ground in to your right foot. Lift your left foot up and cross your left leg over your right knee. Hook your foot behind your right calf. Squeeze your legs together and squat a little bit deeper.

For your arms, reach them out in front of you as if you were going to hug someone. Place the right arm under the left crossing your arms in front of your chest. Bend your elbows so the back of your hands come to touch. Then press the front of your palms together. Gaze at your hands.

Come out of this pose slowly: hands first, then feet. Be sure to do the other side.

To improve the pose:

- Make your lower body smaller by "sitting" and make your upper body longer by lifting your elbows.
- Breathe deep to stay balanced, remembering the six balancing tips.

There are many easier variations of this. Do what feels comfortable:

- Only do your arms.
- Only do your legs.
- Cross your legs not hooking your foot around the calf.
- Hug yourself as opposed to doing the full arm expression of the pose.
- Let the back of the hands touch as opposed to the palms.

Why should I do it?

In this pose, you are slightly crouching as a perched eagle would. Eagles are wise, focused, and poised for action. These characteristics are needed to combat fear!

This pose also:

- Helps develop focus.
- Teaches concentration.
- Strengthens your calf muscles.
- Stretches your hips.
- Relieves tension in your shoulders and shoulder blades.

Dancer Pose
(*Natarajasana*)

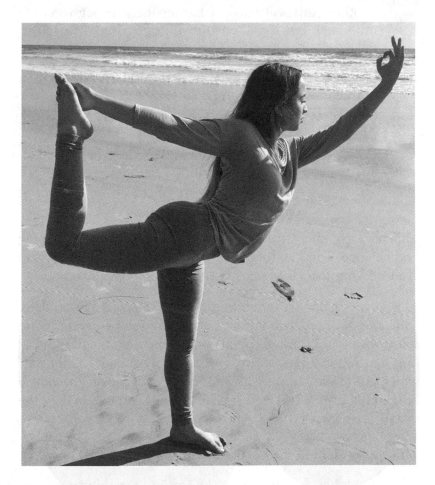

How do I do it?

From Mountain Pose, press strongly into your right foot and begin to lift your left leg up off the ground. Bend your left knee and reach around for your foot using your left hand. Kick back into your hand making a bow shape with your leg. Your chest should begin to "puff out." Reach the right arm out in front of you and then up. The full pose is grabbing your foot (with one or both of your hands) and letting it reach the back of your head

Come out slowly: bring your hand down, then your leg. Be sure to do the second side.

To improve the pose:

- Make sure your hips are straight and in line with one another (this will make it harder for your leg to come up higher, but it will ensure you don't hurt yourself or fall over!).

- Use a strap. Hook it on your foot and have the strap in both hands, helping you backbend here.

- Focus on your breath as it will help when you backbend.

- Press your hand into the wall and use it to help you balance as you go into the pose.

Why should I do it?

This pose combines two very vulnerable poses: heart opening and balance. This can totally be scary. Know that, though, you are free from fear (fear is just a trick our minds play on us).

This pose is named after and represents a special Hindu deity (Shiva or Nataraja) who represents liberation or freedom! He is known as the "Lord of the Dance" and the statue of him has him dancing in a ring of fire, with four arms, on a small dwarf which is the symbol for fear and ignorance. This is the dance of triumph over fear! Let this pose remind you to dance in the face of fear.

This pose also:

- Stretches the muscles in the front of the thigh.

- Strengthens your belly and spine.

- Stretches your shoulders a lot.

- Teaches you balance.

Warrior 3
(*Virabhadrasana 3*)

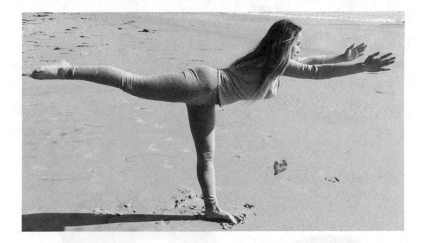

How do I do it?

From Mountain Pose, firmly press your right foot into the ground and kick your left leg back. Reach both of your arms out in front of you and continue to balance forward reaching your arms forward and your leg back. Your hips should be even with one another and your foot flexed. The goal of this pose is to get your legs, back, neck, and arms in one straight line!

Come out slowly with balance and do the same thing on the other side.

To improve the pose:

- Bend your legs if you need to.

- Use the wall: either press your hands or your foot into it for balance.

- Remember the 6 tips for balancing.

- Don't forget to breathe.

Why should I do it?

When you face fear, you have to be a peaceful warrior. Stand strong, find your balance, and look fear right in its eye. With this strength, focus, and control, fear doesn't stand a chance!

This pose is difficult and you may fall out of it: it's ok; let each attempt help you practice facing your fears and take all the lessons this pose provides!

This pose also:

- Builds stomach muscles.

- Teaches endurance.

- Stretches almost all parts of your body.

- Teaches you balance.

- Makes your ankles and feet strong.

Side Plank Pose
(*Vasisthasana*)

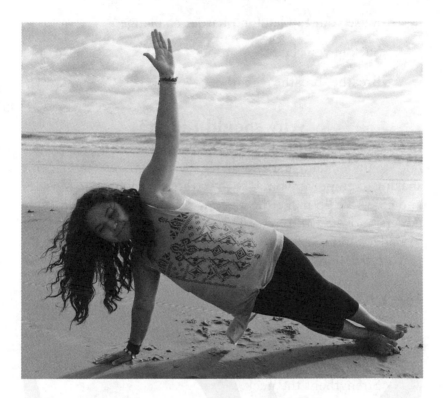

How do I do it?

Come in to a regular plank pose with your body lifted off the ground; be sure your shoulders are in line with your wrists, and your hips with your shoulders, while your legs are stretched out long. Then, place your right hand in the middle of the mat (in line with your left hand). Open your left arm, making your shoulders in line with one another. Stack your feet on top of one another. Stay here as long as you can—challenge yourself. On your exhale, come back to traditional plank, then open up to your other side.

To improve the pose:

- Bring your bottom knee to the ground to help support you.

- Raise your top leg for a harder challenge.

- Suck in your belly.

- Breathe, breathe, breathe.

Why should I do it?

In this pose, most people shake. Shaking is good: it teaches our body to understand fear and then gain strength over it. Use this shaking to empower you. Use the strength in your arm muscles and core to help make the shaking go away. When your body understands how to physically combat fear, the mind will start to understand too. Let this pose remind you of your strength: you are one tough person and fear should be afraid of you.

This pose also:

- Opens the chest.

- Strengthens the ankles.

- Strengthens the neck.

- Teaches balance.

- Helps prepare you for harder arm balances and inversions.

Scale Pose
(*Tolasana*)

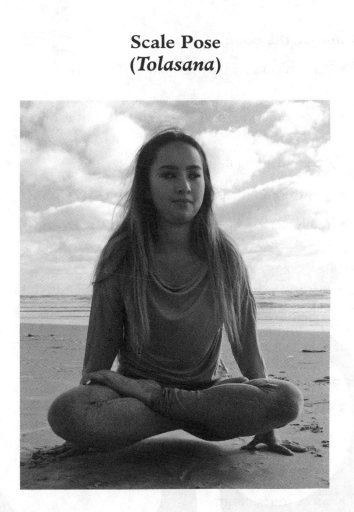

How do I do it?

Sit in Lotus Pose. Bring your hands on the ground next to your hips. Squeeze your shoulder blades together, take a deep inhale and begin to lift off of the ground. Hold here as long as you can. Come down on an exhale. Re-cross the legs the opposite way and repeat the pose.

To improve the pose:

- Place blocks under your hands. This will make it easier to lift up.

- If you can't do Lotus Pose, do Half Lotus or cross your ankles.

- Suck in your belly.

- Breathe and focus on the strength of your arms.

- Really place your palms firmly into the ground.

Why should I do it?

Research shows that this pose helps people with ADD focus better. When there is focus, the mind is not wandering. Most wandering minds, wander right into fear, so a focused mind means a peaceful mind.

This pose also:

- Strengthens your arms, wrists, and hands.

- Makes your belly strong.

- Stretches your hips.

- Gives your energy.

- Teaches you balance and control.

- Helps prepare you for more difficult arm balances and inversions.

Crow/Crane Pose
(*Bakasana*)

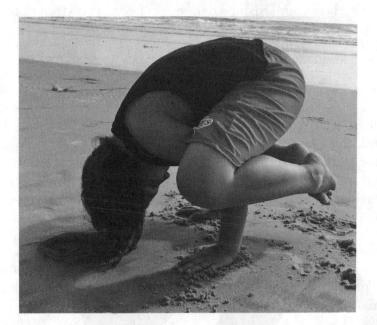

How do I do it?

Come into a squat, and bend forward placing your hands on the floor, shoulder-width apart from one another. Spread your fingers really wide to create a strong and wide base to support your body.

Bend your elbows and slowly lift your heels up off the floor. You're going to shift your body weight forward towards your hands, resting your shins as close to your armpits as possible.

To improve the pose:

- Take your time. Lift one leg up at a time to learn balance.

- If you can't lift up (many people can't as this is very hard and takes a lot of practice) place a block under your forehead and use this to teach you balance as you rest your head but are tipping your body forward.

- Suck your belly in, you need a really strong core to do this pose.

- Have your Dristi be right out in front of you (not down—you'll fall if you look down).

- To make it harder, straighten your arms completely.

Why should I do it?

This pose is named after a graceful animal, the crane. Like the bird, this pose exhibits a lot of grace. It is difficult to do and takes a lot of practice and strength. A lot of times it seems like you are going to fall and smash your face! The truth is, fear is making us think that way. It's actually pretty hard to fall on your face in this pose!

When you are focused, and you don't let fear guide you, you will be graceful, and from this place of grace strength comes! Take your time and keep practicing. I'm still working on doing this one as it truly is a scary pose!

This pose also:

- Strengthens your arms.

- Makes your wrists strong.

- Stretches your back.

- Teaches balance.

- Strengthens your belly.

Breathing

One of the first things you probably stop doing when you are scared is breathing. Watch any scary movie, what do people do when they are scared? Scream (no breathing). Run (barely breathing properly). Gasp (that sound is literally made when you stop breathing!). When you are scared, you have to remember to breathe. This is very difficult because when you are scared, you are not thinking properly (so breathing is probably the last thing on your mind), but practicing breathing every day will help you remember to breathe, when you need it more than ever.

- Notice your breath by placing both of your hands on lungs.

- Breathe in really deep so both of your lungs raise. Try to breathe in through your nose as that's where filtered air comes in.

- On your exhale, release all of the air out through your mouth. Do it dramatically: even make noise doing this!

Note: The focus of this breath is the exhale. The exhale literally cleanses and detoxifies the body. Emotionally, it is important to detoxify yourself from your fears, so let those loud, long exhales represent all the fears that are leaving your mind and body. You should not only feel less scared, but much lighter.

Meditation

There is a really good mudra that you can use that will help you release any fears you are dealing with. It is called the "No Fear" Mudra. Doing this while sitting and meditating (or doing this gesture while doing any of the poses where your hands are free) will absolutely help eliminate fear in your life.

Try it:

- Sit comfortably (you know the drill by now!)

- Lift your right hand above your right thigh and place your palm face out.

- Let your left hand do whatever you want (most people have it rest on the left knee or do Cin Mudra).

- Breathe, and work on clearing your mind.

- Watch the fears drift away.

Writing

Meditative Writing AUMwork 1:

Fear is an ugly little devil trying to stop you from doing what you want to or should do. A lot of people deal with fear by ignoring it, but you can't ignore the devil: it will come back and haunt you until you deal with it. Deal with the devil by using writing. Write down the fears you are dealing with. Just having them down on paper will release them from your mind. Then challenge yourself, how can you alleviate this fear in your life? Come up with a healthy plan to battle the devil known as fear.

Meditative Writing AUMwork 2:

The opposite of fear is inspiration! The fear-devil hates inspired, positive people. Use writing to get you to this place:

- Write about things that inspire you.

- Write about ways to use inspiration to combat any fears you have.

- Be an inspiration. Write about ways to help inspire others to fight the fear in their life.

Chapter 8

Yoga for Confidence

A big, big problem that you might be facing may be with self-confidence. Most teens—boys and girls—have issues with how they feel and think about themselves. If you feel this way, know this is completely normal. Probably most of your peers feel this way, and guess what: I felt this way too.

You may think you are ugly or fat or weird or stupid. You may have heard this because others (bullies) said this to you. You may also feel this way because someone in your life is putting pressure on you to be or look or act a certain way.

A huge problem you may have with confidence can be with school: if you don't get a certain grade on a test or in a subject you might feel really dumb, or if you don't know the answer to a question, you may feel just stupid. They say high school is preparing you for the "real world," and it is important to do well in school so you must work really, really, really hard and that is the first priority. School is important, and you should work hard, but what really prepares you for the real world, more than anything else, is how you deal with your emotions.

Another area that may test your confidence is your appearance. For teenagers, it seems the most important thing can be your appearance. Celebrities, magazines, and television shows sort of dictate what is beautiful. What I wish I knew as a teen was that (1) celebrities are a fake attractive (they are photo-shopped and coved in tons of makeup masking what they really look like), (2) appearances fade, so in the bigger picture of life, it really doesn't matter, and (3) attractiveness is not a fact, but an opinion: everyone is attracted to different people, so many people will think you are attractive and many may not, but none of that matters: what matters is what you think about yourself.

I wish I knew these things when I was your age because I wasted a lot of stress worrying about my appearance: I was tall and gangly for my age and I was a "late bloomer." My boobs never started to grow (I didn't get boobs until I was in college)! I also have these "black dots" on my face; some people called them moles, my mom called them "beauty marks." I hated them and wished I could scratch them off. I also hated my nose and my hair and spent too much time thinking about clothes! I felt like no one would like me or date me and I wished I could be other people.

Teens have a lot of pressures, so I know that just telling you things doesn't make it go away, but know that your body constantly changes, as does your appearance, throughout your entire life. It has to: it's part of the aging process. What you look like today is not what you will look like in a month, a year, a decade and so on, so it really is wasted energy.

Your body is one of the most important things, but what it looks like is not the most important. The most important is how it feels: when you are physically and emotionally healthy, you look good. It's the truth: happy and healthy people are the prettiest people. The fact that you are sitting down, reading a book about a way to be mentally and physically happy and healthy, in my opinion, makes you beautiful already.

Another huge problem you may have is with friends or cliques. If you ever felt like you didn't fit in know most people have felt that way. Making friends can be tough especially when there can be pressures put on you to act or look a certain way, but the good news is there are SO many people in this world. Everyone may not like you (not everyone likes me), but it really doesn't matter as long as you are yourself and believe in yourself. When you gain inner confidence, then you will know you're funny enough, smart enough, pretty enough, _____ (fill in adjective here) enough.

A last huge problem you may have with your confidence is pressure for being the "best." American society is the most competitive society in the world. Marketing's aim is to make you feel unworthy. That, in my opinion, is super sad and manipulative.

For many people, from the time we are little, we are told to be the best and if we aren't working to be the best, we are the worst. I've literally been told second place is the same as last place! Your family, job, sport's team, or anywhere else may make you feel this way. When people tell you this, you start to believe it. As an adult, I've learned competition only hurts people; it is only when we work together and help each other (instead of working against each other) can the best stuff happen. Many countries in this world live this way, so open your mind: being the "best" may just be some concept someone made up, that doesn't really matter or exist.

Competition always gives people a false identity: the people who are characterized the "best" can become conceited or over-confident. When your confidence is over-balanced you have no room to grow and become better learning from others. When there is no growth, you won't stay the best for too long.

I know all of these things because I've been there (I was the young girl looking in the mirror wishing for something else), and I've taught many adults and teens who have felt confused or lost with their own self-confidence. Yoga has helped me so much in realizing that I am beautiful and perfect just as I am, and it has also helped me help others see this too. Stretching, breathing, meditating, and writing will help get you there too (and if you already are confident it will help keep you there!).

Stretches: Inversions

An inversion is a pose where you head is lower than your heart. Inversions help you see the world upside down, literally. When you invert your body, you are flipping yourself upside down and you can physically see the world around you from a new perspective: when you are able to do this, you are able to open your mind and see things more clearly. This will help you realize new and exciting things about yourself and the world. It will make you a more open-minded person. A more open-minded person is more accepted and flexible, which leads to being more successful with love, friends, and school...essentially everything!

Inversions are very difficult. Because they are not easy, they help build confidence: when you are in a headstand, you are going to feel so confident and strong!

Inversions also help you to work on your confidence. Honestly, it's super scary to stand on your head or flip your body upside down: that is not normal for your bodies (what is normal is for you to feel freaked out or weird about it). Let these poses teach you to work on your confidence: try your hardest to not get mad at yourself if you can't do it. There are no such things as failures. Every moment of life is a lesson teaching us to be a better person.

Also, there is no rush with yoga: it is a practice (a practice you do your whole life). There are still lots of poses I can't do, and handstand is one of them. It's all good. I will get there when I can, and in the meantime, I'll keep practicing and work on being a stronger, more confident person both physically and mentally.

Things take time, so take your time. Don't rush. This is how you hurt yourself. Believe in yourself though! If you don't believe in yourself, who will? Confidence starts with you.

Last, don't be a show off! There are some adults in the yoga classes that I teach and take that literally show off their poses. As a yoga teacher, I don't really care if a person can do a hard pose or not. That does not make them a good person. To me, what makes a person a good person is someone who is honest and works on themselves to be confident, loving, grateful, and peaceful (all of the concepts we discussed in this book!).

So, taking a "cool" picture of you doing a hard pose and putting it on Instagram® doesn't guarantee you are a cool person. Just like with adults, what makes you cool is being positive with your emotions and helping others feel good too.

Note: Negative thoughts make us have a heavy mind and energy. The heavier your mind, the harder it will be for you to flip upside down! First, release yourself from all thoughts: forget where you are and focus on your body (the worst thing you can do is think: "I can't do it" You 100% won't be able to do it if you think that way). There is nothing to be scared of in these poses: as long as you follow the directions, and stay focused on the present moment, you will not get hurt.

Plow Pose
(*Halasana*)

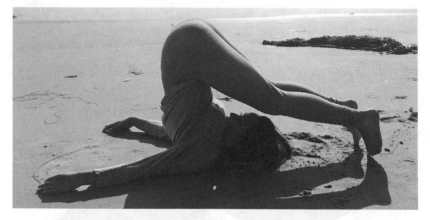

How do I do it?

Laying on your back, take a deep inhale. On your exhale, begin rocking back and forth until eventually your legs come behind your head. Straighten out your legs the best that you can with your feet resting on the ground behind you. Your spine should be totally straight as your neck and shoulders are on the ground. Your hands can come to your lower back or on the ground for support.

To get out of this pose, bend your knees and slowly (vertebrae by vertebrae) bring your spine back flat to the ground. Take a few breaths as you hang out in a neutral place; then, move your body in whatever way feels good.

To improve the pose:

- It is difficult to breathe in this pose because your lungs are flipped over and your air ways are constricted a bit. Breathe consciously here, as it will help you build your lungs' strength along with making the pose easier.
- Press your toenails down into the ground to help straighten your legs.
- Lift your chest towards your chin.
- You can interlace your fingers together and stretch them out behind you for a deeper shoulder stretch.

- If your legs don't come all the way to the ground, it is normal! Bend your knees and hang out wherever it feels good.

Why should I do it?

What is really hard for many people to understand (both adults and teens) is that confidence comes from our own truth within ourselves that helps us define what makes us feel proud about ourselves. Society and conditioning plays a big part in blurring up this definition. The most popular songs on the radio sing about what makes people "cool" or "normal." TV shows, movies, and fashion/marketing play a big role, too, in giving us a pretend definition of what we should be to feel worthy.

It is really hard, and you have to be brave to do this, but when you see through all of this, you will realize that YOU are what makes your own definition of what is "cool" and "normal": not anything or anyone else (and that you are already cool and normal from this definition). Plow Pose helps us flip upside down, get rid of the blurriness, and be brave which helps us see things from their true prospective: inward!

This pose also:

- Stretches your shoulders.

- Helps you sleep better.

- Is good for stomach cramps.

- Helps get rid of headaches.

- Makes your back feel really good.

Shoulderstand
(*Salamba Sarvangasana*)

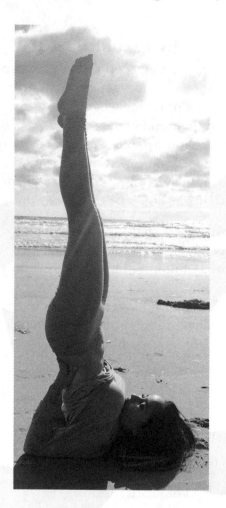

How do I do it?

Plow Pose is a perfect place to get into Shoulderstand. Follow the directions for Plow, then with your hands on the small of your back, start to straighten your legs one at a time. Your legs, hips, and shoulders should be in a straight line. You should be using the strength of your shoulders to hold you as you invert your body here (never use your neck).

Come out of this pose slow: bring the legs down behind you for Plow; then come down vertebrae by vertebrae until everything is straight and neutralized. Hang out here for a few breaths before you move your body.

To improve the pose:

- Point or flex your feet to keep your legs active and strong.

- Breathe deep here as it is much harder to breathe in this position.

- Place a blanket under your shoulders to help make this pose easier and more comfortable.

- Work on really opening your chest here by bringing it closer to your chin.

Why should I do it?

This pose is perfect preparation for the more difficult inverted poses of Headstand, Handstand, and Scorpion Pose. Use this pose to practice understanding what your body feels like upside down! This pose will also help you strengthen your core (which is your energetic spot of confidence!). This will give you the confidence needed to go into the harder inversions!

This pose is often referred to as the "queen" of all poses because you are active yet restorative. Your entire body weight is supported by your upper body. This helps build strength and help you to get comfortable with inverting your body while still being calm. This is the key to gaining self-confidence. Besides, who is more confident than the queen

This pose also:

- Makes you calm: it soothes the nervous system!
- Stretches your neck.
- Strengthens your shoulders.
- Gives you energy.
- Helps with digestion.

Headstand
(*Salamba Sirshasana*)

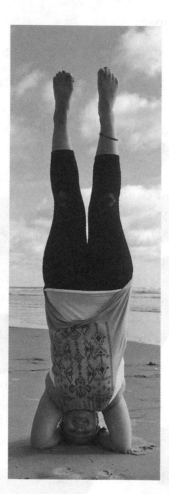

How do I do it?

Interlace your fingers together, then press your forearms into the ground. Your elbows should be in line with your shoulders, Bend forward placing your head on the ground. Your body will look like a Downward Facing Dog only your head and forearms are on the ground. Lift your heels and begin to walk your feet in close to your head. The goal is to get your hips in line with your shoulders. When everything is lined up, bend one knee to your chest and find your balance. Then bring both knees to your chest. Take your time straightening your legs.

To come out of this pose, come slow. Bring your legs slowly down to the floor, and rest in Child's Pose.

To improve the pose:

- Be sure your press your pinky and ring finger, along with your forearms on the ground.

- The forearms and shoulders are supporting most of the weight in your body (not your head).

- Squeeze your legs together to keep yourself inverted and strong.

- If you feel like you are going to fall forward, bend your knees (this will stop you) or tuck your chin into your chest to make your fall more graceful!

- Use the wall behind you or a friend holding your legs to help you with your balance.

- Breathe and believe in yourself!

Why should I do it?

This pose is known as the "king of all yoga poses." The reason for this is it has a lot of physical benefits that are very powerful for your body. In the same, just like a king, to do it, you need to be strong and confident.

This pose also:

- Creates good posture.
- Increases strength in the shoulders, neck, and stomach.
- Improves circulation and energy level.
- Builds your immune system.
- Increases concentration.
- Stimulates pressure points of your head for balance.

Handstand
(*Adho Mukha Vrkshasana*)

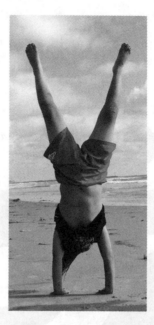

How do I do it?

The secret to Handstand Pose is to pretend your hands are your feet and your feet are your hands. You are flipping your body over: but standing as strong as you do on your hands as you would on your feet in Arms Over Head Pose. To get there:

- Stand facing the wall about two to four feet away from it.

- Place your hands flat on the floor (make sure your wrists are under your shoulders).

- Keep your arms straight and find a Dristi (a spot to look at in between your hands and the wall).

- Kick one leg up at a time.

- Use the wall to help you line your hips up with your hands.

- Come down very slow and mindfully, one leg at a time, resting in Child's Pose.

To improve the pose:

- Rest your feet or foot on the wall and slowly practice removing one or both of them

- Point your toes and squeeze your legs together to stay tight in your core.

- Spread your fingers really wide to have maximum space on the ground.

- Don't arch your back.

- Release heavy (negative thoughts) from your head!

- Breathe.

Why should I do it?

When you are standing on your hands, you can't think of anything but being strong, and strength only comes from confidence. The only way to get into this pose is to have the confidence to do it: everyone has the ability to do this, they just need to dig deep down inside to find that place of self-worth. Dig deep: you got this!

This pose also:

- Makes your arms strong.

- Makes your wrists healthy.

- Releases tension in your shoulders.

- Makes your belly muscles strong.

- Strengthens your spine.

Scorpion Pose
(*Pincha Mayurasana*)

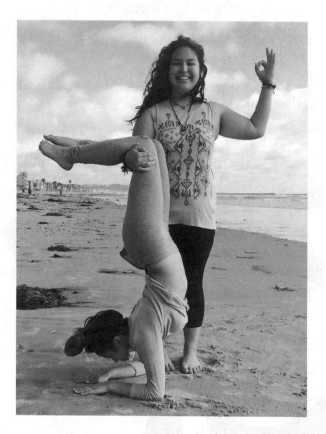

How do I do it?

From Downward Dog, bring your forearms to the ground. Your palms should be flat against the floor (just like your feet would be if you were standing upright). Press your elbows firmly in the ground. Squeeze your shoulders in the direction of your hips (this will help you expand your chest which will help you balance).

Walk your feet in. Press through your arms. Stretch your neck long. Kick high (one leg at a time), and when both of your legs are upright, start to bend your knees. Keep back bending here as the more you bend your knees, reaching your toes towards your head and your head towards your feet, the more likely you will stay balanced.

To improve the pose:

- Place a block in between your hands to help understand where your arms should be positioned.

- Balance your feet on a wall.

- Have your friend or teacher spot you: either holding your legs or having your knees bend over their arm.

- Have your gaze be in front of your hands.

Why should I do it?

This pose is named after a peacock feather because it resembles a peacock with its tail feather spread striving to get the attention of others! Let this pose remind you: all things are the same. When a peacock is spreading its feathers, it is beautiful and confident, and all notice it! Spread your feathers too! The world wants to notice you, for you are beautiful (we all are).

This pose also:

- Stretches the shoulders.
- Strengthens the upper back.
- Makes your back and shoulders very flexible.
- Tones your stomach.

Breathing

As you know, when we breathe, we inhale and exhale. The inhales and exhales have very powerful jobs.

The inhales physically nurture the body: it feeds our body more throughout the day than food does! Emotionally, the inhale helps feed our confidence and inspiration. As we breathe in deep, our inhales fulfill us, helping us feel complete and worthy.

As we talked about, the exhale cleanses us. For this breathing exercise we are going to invite inspiration in to our emotional body while releasing anything emotionally holding us back from feeling confident enough to do so. We are going to do this physically by using the breath.

Here's how:

- Whenever you are ready, take the deepest inhale you can. Feel your body feel completely full of inspiration! Let this feeling remind you of all the good that is within you and that you have to share with the world.

- When you feel you are ready to exhale, picture all the negativity that holds you back from seeing the amazingness you possess. Exhale all of this, removing it from your body.

- Continue to breathe in this way to help build your confidence.

Meditating

True confidence comes from a place where you see far deeper than your physical self: this allows you to realize that beauty is much more than appearance; it has to do with your insides. To "see" your insides, try meditating with a mirror:

- Sit or stand in front of a mirror.

- First look at your entire body from head to toe (Tell all the judging and any negative thoughts your brain has on your physical appearance to be quiet).

- Then focus on your eyes. Stare at your eyes in the mirror.

Stare deeper, way past their color: What do you see? Who are you?

- Look away by blinking your eyes closed, and then notice, what do you see when you are not physically looking at your body anymore but you are looking inward?

- Reflect on your experience. This person you saw: this is the true you, and this person is beautiful. This is absolutely something to confident about.

Note: If it is hard for you to look in the mirror, don't worry. Many people have this issue too. Take your time.

Writing

Meditative Writing AUMwork 1:
Everyone has at least one thing that they like or they are good at: this thing is known as their dharma (or their destiny). You can't fight destiny, so whatever it is you are good at or whatever experiences you are going through now are preparing you for the job you will have and the impact you will make on the world.

Think about what you really like doing. You don't have to figure out everything right now (I sure didn't when I was your age: I changed my major 3 times in college, and now I am doing something indirectly related to my degrees). Start to write about it. Also, think about what stuff plays a big part in your life (even if it is negative); this can play a part in helping you fulfill your dharma. There is purpose to everything.

My anxiety and depression led me to where I am today. If I wasn't so nervous growing up, I wouldn't be the calm adult I am today, teaching yoga and helping other nervous people feel better too. This gives me confidence about all the negative fear I faced in my life.

Think about all of these things, and then write down all of your thoughts.

Meditative Writing AUMwork 2
If you're feeling not confident enough:
Create a list of all the things that you like about yourself. Keep this list. Try to add at least one characteristic about yourself that you like to the list whenever you can. Keep adding until you have pages and pages. Read this list when you are feeling not very confident.

Meditative Writing AUMwork 3:
If you're feeling overconfident:
Write down a list of all the things you still want to and need to learn. What don't you know yet? Sometimes when people are overconfident they feel like they are "know-it-alls." Nobody knows it all and everyone can benefit from learning every day, so what else can you learn? Let this information humble you, and then inspire you. Go out and learn something new (and don't worry about being the best at this new topic; just take in the new information to make you a smarter and better person).

When I was a teen, I was very insecure about the way I looked, yet I did not want anyone to know that I had a poor self-image because I didn't want people to think of me as "insecure." I wanted people to think I was confident and had it all together, so I pretended to be happy, feel confident, and not care about the way I looked. But behind closed doors I was worried about who didn't like me and what others thought about me.

I lost a bunch of weight and was obsessed with my looks in order to feel better about myself. Lucky for me, it never worked. I never found that I actually felt better about myself when I was thinner. It wasn't until I was able to look at the deeper issues I was feeling about who I was as a person (I thought I was not enough as I was) and heal them, that I finally found peace and joy in my life.

As an adult, I look back at all the years I spent struggling to try and maintain an image, covering up how I truly felt deep down. If I would have had the courage to let someone in and share how I was really feeling, I may have been able to receive some support. This could have saved me 20 years of an eating disorder!

I have learned that all humans have places inside that are tender and need extra support. Today I have grown to love those places within and have been able to heal my misunderstandings about my worth and value and now have the honor of helping others do the same.

—Lesley, 34

Chapter 9

AUM

Today I saw a little baby bird's nest. It was not any bigger than a quarter. In there, there was a little, little baby egg. Here I saw AUM.

This nest and bird family is not any different than us: human beings. The mama bird, although small, used her love and the power it gave her, to build a nest for her offspring to rest, be born, and live until it left to start its own life. I'm sure this wasn't easy for her, but just by looking at this nest, I could tell it was built from love. Isn't this what those who take care of us do for us? They try their best, using the power of their love, to give you, their offspring, a place to rest, be born and live until it's time for you to start a life of your own.

AUM is the sacred sound chanted or sang in yoga. Try it: take a deep inhale, and on your exhale say Aaa—uuuuu—-mmmmmm (close your lips on the "mmmm" part.) Weird at first, but its nice, right? You will see: the more you hear it, chant it, and say it, the more comforting it will make you feel.

AUM has been translated in many ways, but all of these translations relate to one thing: the belief that we are all the same. The best definition I have ever heard of AUM is that its the sound made when every person in the world says their name at exactly the same time. It is the sound of the world. Think about that. It is the sound of oneness.

Have you ever heard someone be described as "having a good heart deep down inside?" I've heard so many people say: "He really has a good heart underneath it all." or "She really is a good person deep down." This is because we all are love.

Everyone deserves love, and everyone wants love (even if they won't admit it). It is a birthright of ours to love and be loved.

Negative emotions like fear, anger, impatience, sadness, jealously, obsession, worry, lack of appreciation, and lack of focus really blur us from remembering what we are: love! Some of us show AUM clearly (like Martin Luther King Jr., while others have it buried deep down inside like Hitler).

Yoga and AUM reminds us that everyone is love: everyone is the same. Even that really mean kid on your bus. Even the people who started wars and murdered many unrightfully in our history.

AUM takes this explanation of oneness even deeper; AUM does not discriminate: the birds (and their tiny nests), the ocean, the trees, and the sun: all things (living and nonliving) are the same. We all are love.

This may be a big concept to understand, but don't worry you have your whole life to practice it. Whenever you feel negative, I encourage you to see and hear the AUM. Not literally, but symbolically. The bully talking bad about someone is just yearning for love. The jealous friend starting trouble is looking for love too.

It is just not being expressed properly because it hasn't been learned yet. Teach by example. Be AUM

AUM is a really big concept: even its symbol represents oneness, because AUM or oneness exists in our mind. From this prospective, AUM is the mind.

Here is the symbol:
Dylan Age 11

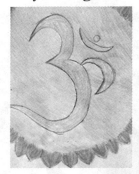

The **top curve** represents the state of sleep. The **bottom and largest curve** represents being awake. The **middle curve** (between the curves representing sleeping and waking) is the dream state. The **curved line under the dot** represents illusion (which is caused by all of those negative emotions that get in the way of love). The **dot** represents the Absolute State: the realization of sameness and love!

I remember one time when I was in high school. I was a senior and there was a freshman on the tennis team I played on (this freshman was also the younger sister of my friend). There was a school dance for freshman and sophomores, and she didn't have a boyfriend to go with, but she wanted to go. The rule was you couldn't go without a date. Since she didn't have a date, I went with her! Lots of people made fun of her and called her gay (oddly, they didn't call me gay: I guess that's because I was a "cool" senior). Regardless, we had a lot of fun, and we went together for this reason: it was nothing sexual; it was all for the sake of love! This is AUM. Calling people gay or making fun of others because they do something different is not.

Where can you find the AUM in your life? Where can you see it? Put your hands over your ears and start to hear that light hum. Hear it? That is AUM. Now listen to a dog barking or an alarm go off, that is AUM: even if the sound is ugly, AUM still exists. Can you hear it?

Practice seeing everyone and everything the same. Look for AUM everywhere (especially in your mind).

About the Author:

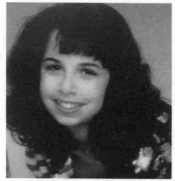 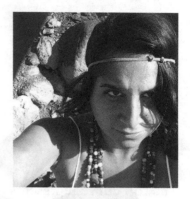

Shawna age 13

Shawna is a San Diego yoga teacher, Reiki master, author, and spiritual activist leading classes, workshops, teacher trainings, retreats, and festivals throughout North America. She has created teacher trainings and authored a number of books. She is the founder of Yin-Reiki, Chakra Camp, and Project Breath—all yogic practices and communities centered on finding bliss through peace, and has created the first ever Yoga Teacher Training for Teens to teach teens to be yoga teachers for other teens! She has a Master in Writing Arts and BA's in Sociology and Early Childhood Education.

Learn more about Shawna at: www.yogawithshawna.com and facebook.com/shawna.schenk or send her an email at: info@yogawithshawna.com and follow her at @San_Diego_Yoga.

Yoga For Teens
Teacher Training

The Yoga For Teens Teacher Training is an 8-week, once a week or one week, 7-day intensive teacher training, offered by Shawna Schenk, to tweens and teens ages 11 to 17. It is open to all boys and girls who want to learn how to use yoga to cope with the different emotions they face on a daily basis. The training provides an easy-to-understand explanation of the deep history of yoga while teaching many of the different yoga positions, breathing techniques and meditation exercises. This information is explained so that teens and tweens can use it in their everyday, modern life while dealing with different emotions including love, anger, fear, patience, focus, peace, and sadness. Then, the tweens and teens learn how to pass this knowledge on to other teens and tweens by leading yoga classes. At the end of the training, the teen/tween is a certified Teen Yoga instructor.

The training encourages teens to bring yoga to all communities for free and use their teachings to promote health and wellness and raise awareness of the importance of handling emotions in a healthy way. Many of the graduated teen and tween teachers have provided classes to raise money to give other teens scholarships to this program for teens and tweens who cannot afford the training, or collect money to provide yoga supplies and books to other teens and tweens so they can learn and practice too.

To have a Teen Yoga Teacher Training in your area, get certified to be a Teen Yoga Teacher or if you are an adult and want to get certified to lead a Teen Yoga Teacher Training or to donate to a scholarship for a teen who cannot afford the training contact Shawna at: info@yogawithshawna.com

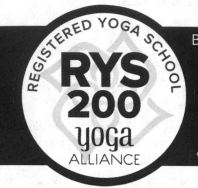

Become a registered yoga teacher (200-hours) through the Yoga Allaince in Yoga With Shawna's 6-month, 9-week, or 2-week intensive training. This training is open to anyone over the age of 12 and is perfect for Mothers and daughtesrs to do together!

The training covers:

- Asana, pranayama, kriyas, chanting, mantra, mudra and meditation

- Yoga philosophies, yoga life style and ethics for yoga teacher

- Human physical anatomy and physiology (bodily organ, etc)

- Energy anatomy and physiology (chakras, nadis, etc.)

- Yoga teaching methodology (including demonstration, observation, assisting, correcting, and adjusting)

- Common issues and proper use of props

- Aryvedia

- Savasana techniques including aromatherapy, Thai massage and Reiki

- The Yoga Sutras, The Pradipika, and The Gitta

- Various yoga styles including: Yin Yoga, Ashantga, Pre-Natal, Kundalini, Iyengar, Acro-Yoga

- The five elements

- Malas, mandalas and other Indian traditions

Contact Shawna at *info@yogawithshawna.com* to inquire about the next training.

Become a Reiki Practioner and study energy in a level 1, 2, or Master's study program. Classes can be online or in person in San Diego.

First Degree Reiki:
Heal your self. (6 hours)

- Private Reiki healing session
- History/linage of Reiki class
- Hands-on training workshop

Second Degree Reiki:
Heal others. (6 hours)

- Attunement Ceremony
- Hands-on Healing Clinic
- Business of Reiki Class

Master Degree:
Train others. (12 month commitment)

- Learn how to train other teachers
- Attunement Ceremony
- Master Symbols

Reiki classes are open to anyone over the age of 7. Contact: info@yogawithshawna.com to take a training.

Enchanting Beauty

Dr. Manisha Kshirsagar, BAMS with Megan M. Murphy, CAP

ISBN: 978-0-9406-7633-6 | Item# 990685 | $19.95 | 310 pp pb

"With flowing prose of wisdom Dr. Kshirsagar unfolds the Vedic secrets of women's health and beauty one flower petal at a time revealing from the inside out the most enchanted life journey for women."
DR. JOHN DOUILLARD
Best Selling Author
LifeSpa.com

"Dr. Manisha Kshirsagar brings her vast knowledge of Ayurvedic medicine together with her expertise as an esthetician to give us the foundation for beauty that radiates from the inside out."
MARCI SHIMOFF
Professional Speaker #1 NY Times Bestselling Author of Happy for No Reason, Love For No Reason, Chicken Soup for the Woman's Soul

"Enchanting Beauty gives readers a refreshing, holistic perspective on the true nature of beauty. Using the wisdom of Ayurvedic medicine and philosophy, as well as personal and professional experience..."
SHEILA PATEL MD
Medical Director,
Chopra Center

"Dr. Manisha Kshirsagar's Enchanting Beauty teaches us the real definition of true beauty- a largely misunderstood concept in modern society. It is an empowering, inspiring work that will enable every woman that reads it to be more in touch with the unique beauty that is her birthright."
Enchanting Beauty by Dr. Manisha Kshirsagar is an excellent Ayurvedic guidebook for promoting inner and outer beauty, happiness and health for women of all ages.
KIMBERLY SNYDER CN
New York Times
Bestselling Author of
The Beauty Detox Solution and The Beauty Detox Power

It is an important addition to the existing Ayurvedic literature and adds much new information and insight in an easy accessible form.
DR. DAVID FRAWLEY

available at bookstores and natural food stores nationwide or order your copy directly by sending cost of item plus $2.50 shipping/handling
75 s/h for each additional copy ordered at the same time) to:

Lotus Press, PO Box 325, Twin Lakes, WI 53181 USA toll free order line: 800 824 6396 • office phone: 262 889 856
office fax: 262 889 2461 email: lotuspress@lotuspress.com • web site: www.lotuspress.com

Lotus Press is the publisher of a wide range of books and software in the field of alternative health, including
Ayurveda, Chinese medicine, herbology, aromatherapy, Reiki and energetic healing modalities. Request our free book catalog.

Yoga Therapy For Health and Healing
Remo Rittiner
ISBN: 978-0-9409-8514-8 | Item# 990660 | $19.95 | 198 pp

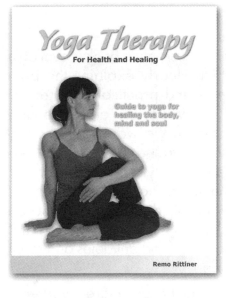

This book is based on the fundamental principles of the yoga tradition according to the yoga master, T. Krishnamacharya and his pupil, A.G. Mohan, and on the latest insights in the study of western anatomy.

It is written in a way that is clear and easy to understand and is suitable for beginners and advanced yoga practitioners alike, who are interested in the great healing potential of yoga therapy. In this book, Remo Rittiner has incorporated his many years of experience with a host of people who regularly practise under his yoga instruction.

- Bestselling Yoga Therapy title from Germany
- Combines Yoga Therapy with Ayurveda For Optimum Results
- Fully Illustrated to Guide Your Application of the Yoga Poses
- Suitable for Individuals For Self-Help As Well As Health Care Practitioners and Physical Therapists
- Specific Practices to Enhance Wellness Such as Stress Reduction and Relaxation

- Addresses Chronic and Acute Health Issues With Specific Yoga Therapies such as Blood Pressure, Back Pain, Neck & Shoulders, Digestion, Asthma, Weight Loss and Obesity, and many more
- Includes Extensive Index of Yoga Asanas (Poses) and a General Index for Ease of Use

Available at bookstores and natural food stores nationwide or order your copy directly by sending cost of item plus $2.50 shipping/handling ($.75 s/h for each additional copy ordered at the same time) to:

Lotus Press, PO Box 325, Twin Lakes, WI 53181 USA toll free order line: 800 824 6396 • office phone: 262 889 856
office fax: 262 889 2461 email: lotuspress@lotuspress.com • web site: www.lotuspress.com

Lotus Press is the publisher of a wide range of books and software in the field of alternative health, including
Ayurveda, Chinese medicine, herbology, aromatherapy, Reiki and energetic healing modalities. Request our free book catalog.

Ayurveda: Science of Self-Healing
Dr. Vasant Lad
ISBN: 9780914955009 | Item# 990120 | $10.95 | 175 pp

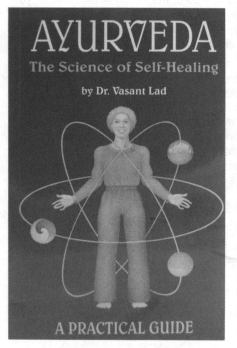

For the first time a book is available which clearly explains the principles and practical applications of ayurveda, the oldest healing system in the world. This beautifully illustrated text throughly explains history & philosophy, basic principles, diagnostic techniques, treatment, diet, medicinal usage of kitchen herbs & spices, first aid, food aid, food antidotes and much more.

Dr.Lad, the premiere ayurvedic practitioner in the U.S.A., clearly explains the principles and practical applications of ayurveda,the oldest healing system in the world. More than 50 concise charts,diagrams and tables are included,as well as a glossary and index in order to further clarify the text.

Available at bookstores and natural food stores nationwide or order your copy directly by sending cost of item plus $2.50 shipping/handling ($.75 s/h for each additional copy ordered at the same time) to:

Lotus Press, PO Box 325, Twin Lakes, WI 53181 USA toll free order line: 800 824 6396 • office phone: 262 889 856
office fax: 262 889 2461 email: lotuspress@lotuspress.com • web site: www.lotuspress.com

Lotus Press is the publisher of a wide range of books and software in the field of alternative health, including
Ayurveda, Chinese medicine, herbology, aromatherapy, Reiki and energetic healing modalities. Request our free book catalog.